One Dish Four Ways

Delicious Low Carb Recipes

57 low-carb recipes and over 100 photos
Packed full of flavour and fantastic exciting meals for everyone

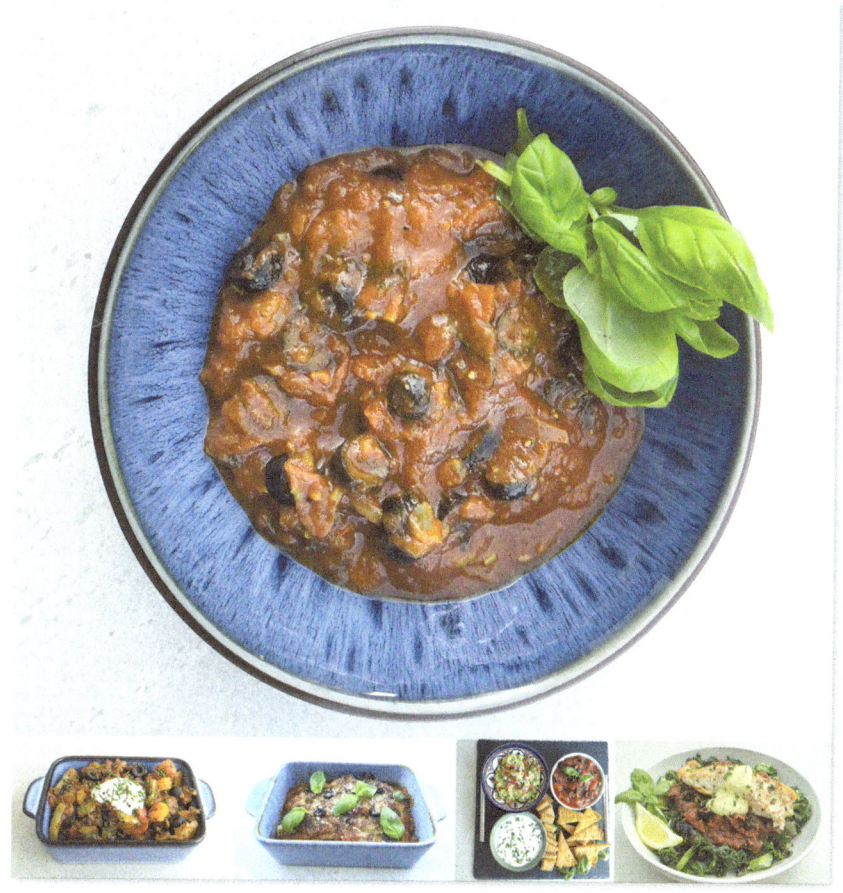

Michele Cooper

"YOU ARE WHAT YOU EAT"

Copyright © 2025 Michele Cooper

All rights reserved. No part of this publication may be reproduced or transmitted in any form or by any means, electronic or mechanical including photocopying, recording or any information storage or retrieval system, without prior permission in writing from the publishers.

The right of Michele Cooper to be identified as the author of this work has been asserted by her in accordance with the Copyright, Designs and Patents Act 1988

First published in the United Kingdom in 2025 by
The Choir Press

ISBN 978-1-78963-410-5

Contents

About One Dish Four Ways   ix
My Family   x
Substitutions   xiii
Thank You   xiv
My Kitchen Gadgets   xv

One Bolognese Four Ways 2

Baked Enchiladas 4
Chilli Bake 6
Cottage Pie 8
Lasagne 10

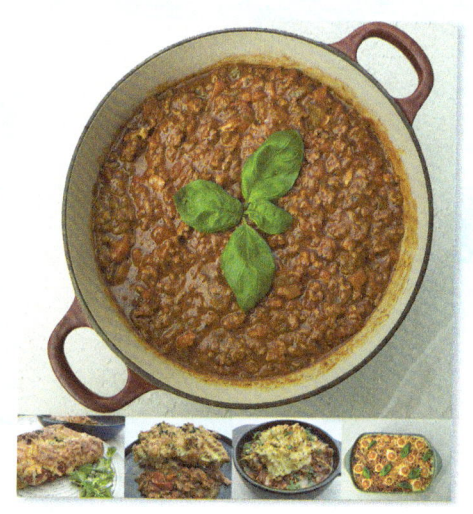

One Coleslaw Four Ways 12

Basil, Sun-dried Tomatoes and Feta 14
Cheddar and Peanuts 15
Curried Eggs 16
Stilton and Walnut, and Optional Apple 17

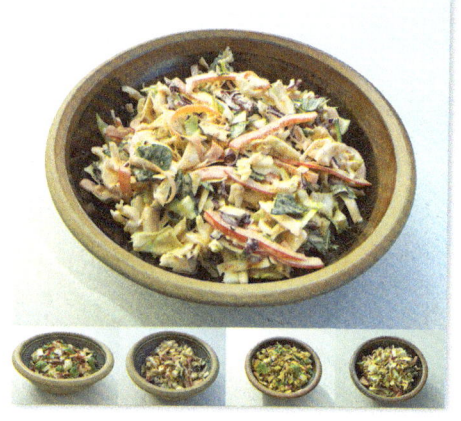

One Crustless Quiche Four Ways 18

Ham and Spring Onion 20
Salmon, Broccoli and Dill 21
Stilton and Mushroom 22
Sundried Tomatoes, Feta and Spinach 23

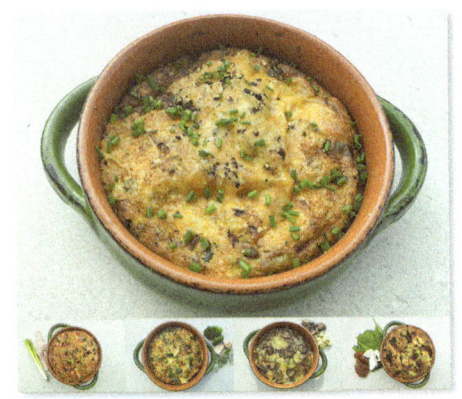

One Curry Four Ways 24

Biryani 26
Chicken and Roast Pepper Curry 28
Roasted Vegetable and Butter Bean Curry 29
Chicken, Tomato and Roasted Vegetable Curry 30

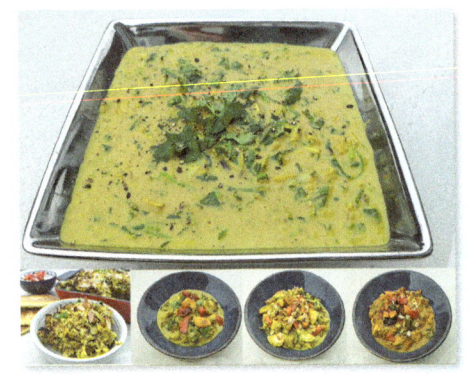

One Pie Crust Four Ways 32

Beef and Leek in Gravy Pie 34
Chicken and Vegetable in Gravy Pie 36
Creamy Chicken and Ham Pie 38
Spinach and Feta Pie 40

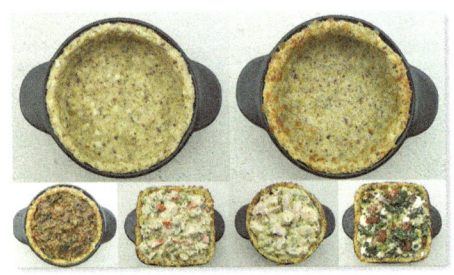

One Rainbow Rice Four Ways 42

Chicken and Chorizo 44
Fish Paella 46
Kedgeree 48
Nutty Vegetarian 50

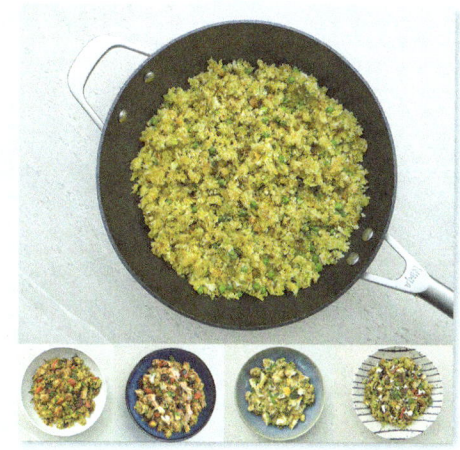

One Salsa Four Ways 52

Baked Vegetables and Chorizo 54
Chicken and Parmesan 56
Salmon and Green Vegetable Parcel 58
Tortilla Chips and 3 Mexican Dips 60

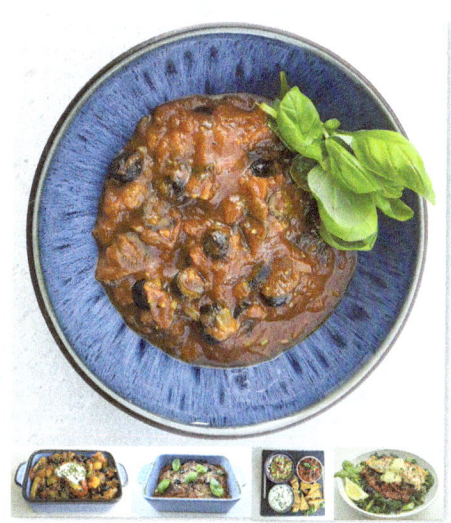

One Soup Four Ways 62

Chicken and Egg Soup 64
Chowder Soup 66
Minestrone Soup 68
Vegetable Smooth and Creamy Soup 70

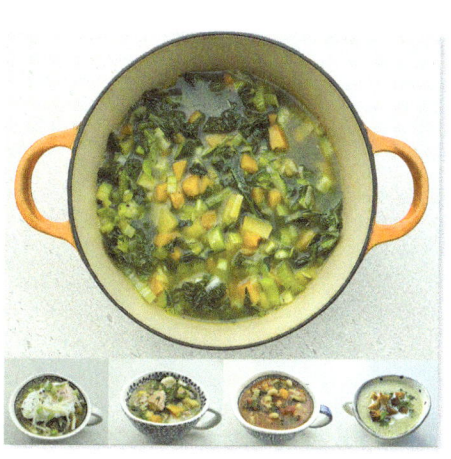

One Yorkshire Pudding Four Ways 72

Lamb and Leek 74

Meatballs in a Tomato Sauce 76

Pesto and Goats Cheese 78

Raspberry Popover 80

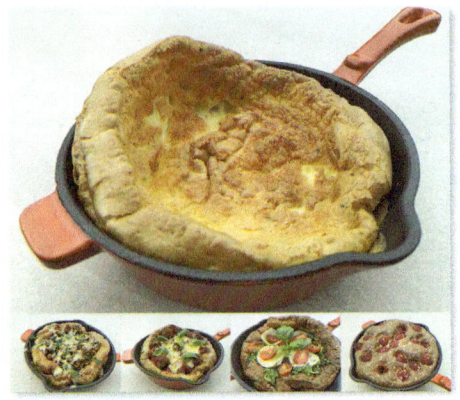

One Custard Tart Four Ways 82

Far Breton 84

Festive Apple Crunch 86

Glazed Fruit Tart 88

Manchester Tart 90

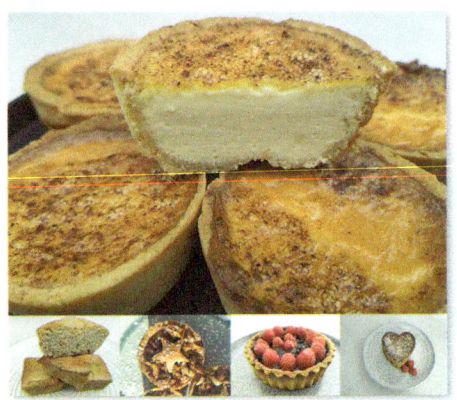

Wraps and Sauces 92

Bamboo Wraps 94

Lupin Wraps 96

MKD (Michele's Keto Dough) 98

Pesto 100

Mayonnaise 102

Tomato Sauce 104

Will's Chilli Oil 106

Index 108

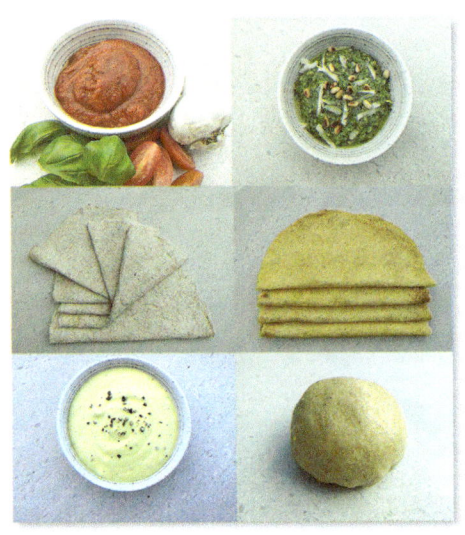

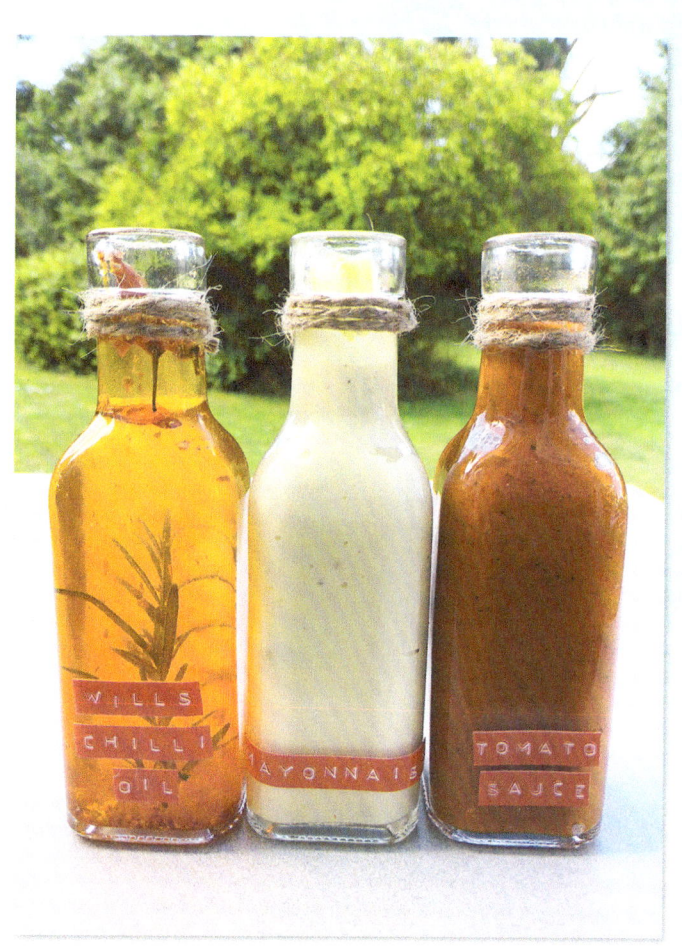

About One Dish Four Ways

About My Book

This book is all about really well-seasoned, nutrient-dense, low-carb base recipes. The base recipes then spin off into four other fabulous recipes.

One Dish Four Ways

In some of these recipes there are a lot of ingredients, but it might just be because they have a lot of store-cupboard ingredients, spices and seasoning. Do not fear the long list!

I am extremely proud of these recipes, and I do hope you'll find you don't need to be low carb to enjoy cooking, eating and sharing these meals with your family and friends.

Originally, I wrote these recipes for my private cookery classes for batch cooking. Each week we would make about 20 portions of meals for the freezer. A lot of washing up was reported, so all my students would come to my online classes with the dishwasher empty! But on the plus side, we finished with a freezer full of fabulous meals for the week.

All the recipes have macros, but the macros may vary depending on where you buy your ingredients from. This is purely a guide.

Carbs / Protein / Calories / Fat

How to Use This Book

I'll try to keep it simple, but once you've made one, it'll all make sense.

1. Choose your recipe. (Every recipe points you back to the base recipe. They are all well labelled with page numbers to guide you.)
2. You'll need the base recipe ingredients.
3. And you'll need the ingredients for the chosen recipe.
4. Once you have all the ingredients, just follow the method in the chosen recipe and the base.
5. And that's it.
6. Enjoy. ♥

My Family

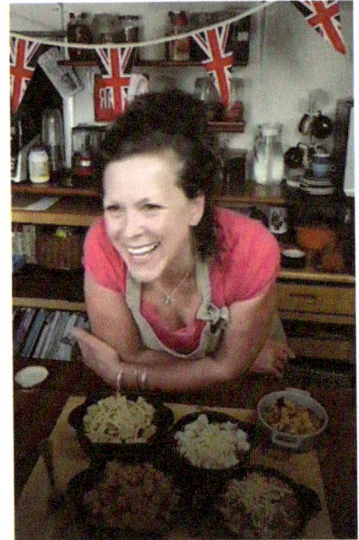
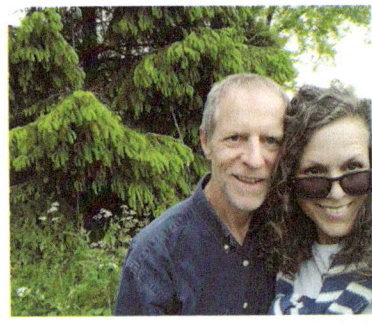
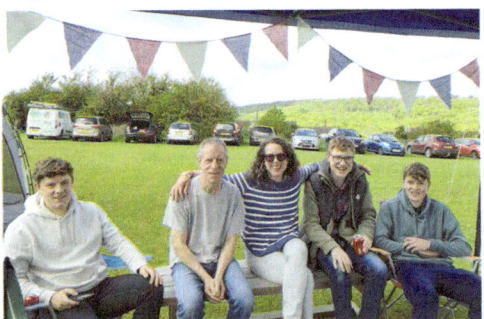
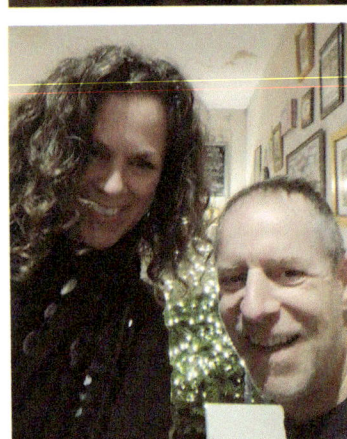
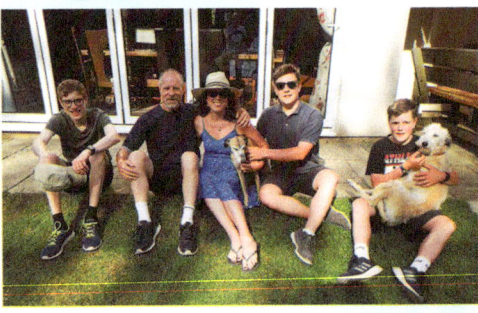
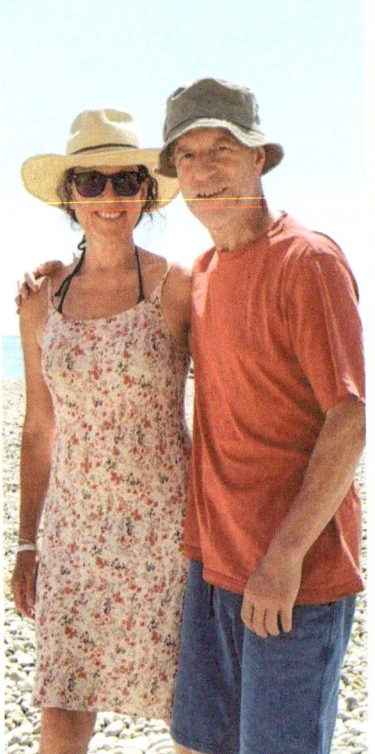
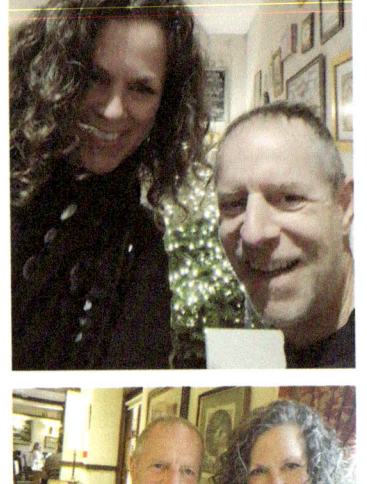
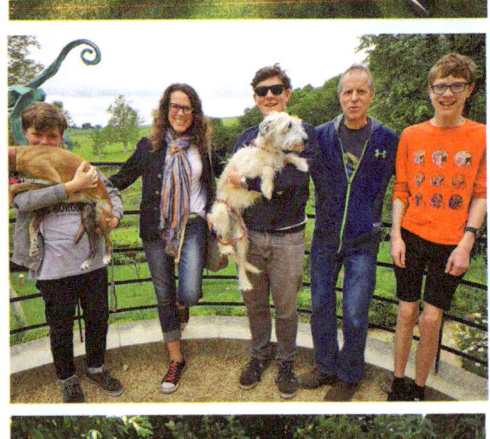
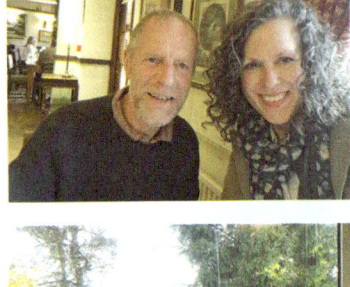
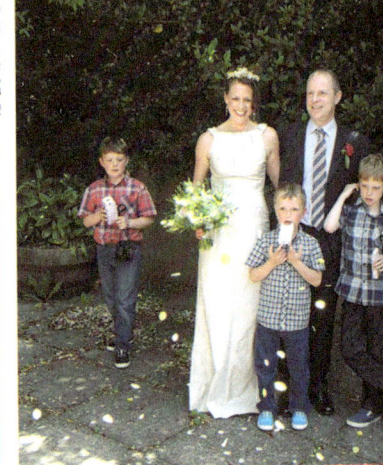
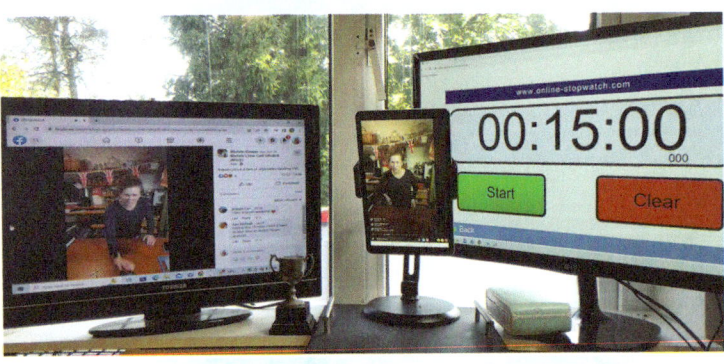

A Little Bit About Our Story

It all started back in 2000, when Peter and I met on holiday in the Dominican Republic. Yes, a holiday romance! William came along the following year, with Freddie and Ollie in quick succession.

Peter and I finally married in 2012. A hot sunny May day, made even more special because the boys were able to be involved, with William reading a poem, Freddie playing his guitar and Ollie being the ring bearer.

Fast forward to July 2016, and, having limped around for many months, Peter was diagnosed with early onset Parkinson's disease. This was an enormous shock for us all. We had to immediately reassess our future, and Peter and I spent time investigating what we could do to support his condition. We were clear that we had to change his diet to maximise his energy levels and reduce well-known inflammation triggers. Parkinson's is currently an incurable illness, but we were determined to do what we could ourselves to keep us as healthy as possible.

In March 2023 we faced a further shock when Freddie was diagnosed with juvenile myoclonic epilepsy. He was away at university at the time and had been suffering regular mini jumps. He had struggled bravely until one day he suffered a collapse while on a video call to us and was admitted to A & E. Thankfully, his condition is now stable, with medication, and at the time of writing he has just started his final year back at university.

The low-carb story

I have been a serial dieter for over 30 years and I have tried many fads along the way. During that time, low carb has featured as the one constant, but with Peter's diagnosis it seemed like the right time to look at this more seriously once again. Initially, we went a bit further and we dabbled with the keto diet, but as those who have tried will know, keto is very hard to sustain, and in any event, Peter began to lose too much weight, and slowly we had to reintroduce more carbs to deal with his particular situation. This led us to where we are now: happy and comfortable with a low-carb and low-GI lifestyle.

I absolutely love creating and adapting traditional recipes to become low carb, and I had an enormous amount of fun putting these recipes together. I can only apologise for some of the portion sizes; I do have four hungry boys!

This book isn't about explaining the science behind eating low carb, but is more about showing you a selection of recipes that I love cooking for my family. I hope it will also play a small part in raising awareness for Parkinson's disease and epilepsy along the way.

I have always been passionate about food, and of course eating! I know from my own experience that food affects the way we feel both physically and mentally. Low carb needn't mean missing out and doesn't have to be boring, and I hope this book will give you some inspiration and confidence to cook everyday meals that everyone can enjoy.

As everybody knows, diet is such an important part of enjoying a healthy lifestyle. I hope this book will prove to be a useful guide in making changes easier and perhaps point you in a better direction, while having some tasty food along the way.

Enjoy! ♥

Substitutions

Throughout the book you'll see a whole range of low-carb vegetables being used in the recipes. Please don't feel you have to stick to the recipe and my choices. Have fun, adapt and use whatever low-carb vegetables you have in the fridge.

For example, in the mash topping (page 8), instead of the cauliflower and swede, you could use celeriac, broccoli, sweet potato, and much more, as long as you cook it well and then blitz it until smooth. The same goes for the rainbow rice (page 42); as long as the main vegetable is predominantly a hard vegetable, like cabbage, cauliflower, swede, celeriac, etc, you can add all sorts of other vegetables to it, like mushrooms, peppers and tomatoes. Have a play; you'll find it's a great way of using up old vegetables.

Thank You

Firstly, I would like to thank Peter and my boys—William, Freddie and Ollie—not forgetting my girls–Cookie and Scoot and Frankie our new family member—for their continual support and entertainment in so many different ways.

Secondly, I would like to thank all my friends who have encouraged, supported and generally really pushed me to write my book. You know who you are. ♥

Thirdly, I would like to thank my book publisher, The Choir Press, for their understanding and for generally looking after me with patience.

And, finally, I would like to thank you for buying and reading this book. I hope it makes sense and that you love the recipes as much as we do.

My Kitchen Gadgets

You'll need your standard kitchen equipment for these recipes, nothing special, **but** if you particularly like the wraps, for example, that appear in some of the recipes, I've explained below why these are a brilliant investment you can use them for.

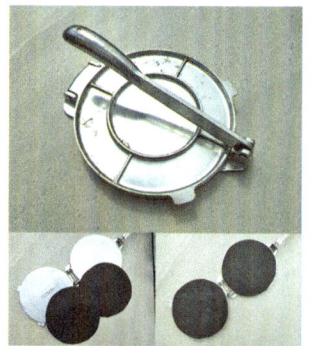

Tortilla Press

These are great for all sorts of dough balls. Whether it's the wrap recipe or you're about to make pizzas, this pushes the dough into an almost perfect circle.

The black circles are oven-liner sheets cut to the shape of the press. If you grease these with olive oil, the dough will slide easily when you press it. These are reusable and last for years.

What to Use if You Don't Have a Tortilla Press
If you don't have a tortilla press, you'll need greaseproof (or silicone) paper, olive oil and a rolling pin.

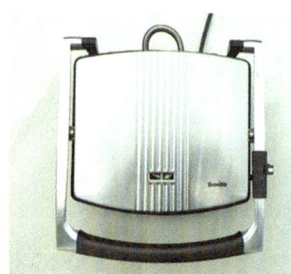

Breville VST026 Four-Portion Sandwich and Panini Press (not sponsored, I just love it)

This compliments the tortilla press beautifully. It will give you the most perfect wraps (page 92)—after you've had a little play—speeding up your prepping and cooking time. You can also use it to par bake or completely cook pizza bases (without the toppings), bake easy tortilla chips, cook perfect Scotch pancakes and cook an English breakfast. And, of course, you can cook panini's in there too!

What to Use if You Don't Have a Panini Press
You can use any other brand—as long as it has flat plates and no ridges—or a good non-stick frying pan, and a little extra time and patience.

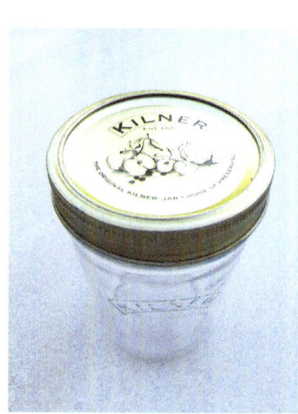

Kilner Jars

These Kilner jars are really useful to have in the cupboard for all sorts of reasons. I particularly like these so I can make the mayonnaise directly in the jar, which saves on time, wastage and washing up.

For sauces and jams, I buy the 350 ml jar, because the end of my hand blender fits perfectly into the base of the jar.

What to Use if You Don't Have Kilner Jars
You can recycle any glass jars with lids.

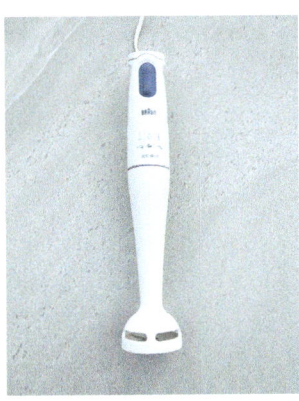

Hand Blender

I mainly use this for making my mayonnaise, mixing it directly in the Kilner jar. Making it this way has a 100% success rate for me. It also has many other uses, like saving a sauce or custard that has gone lumpy.

What to Use if You Don't Have a Hand Blender
For the mayonnaise (page 102) I wouldn't use anything else, but you can use a food processor, although I do get mixed results.

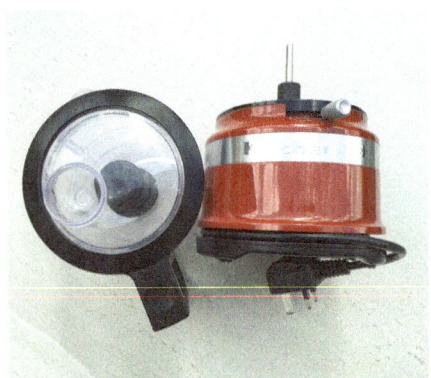

Kitchen Aid Mini Chopper 830 ml

Absolutely any food processor will do, but this is my favourite. It may be small, but it's super versatile and great to have in the kitchen. Once you have it, you'll find lots of uses for it.

What to Use if You Don't Have a Food Processor
It depends what you are using it for, but if it's the rainbow rice (page 42), a sharp knife or grater and patience will do.

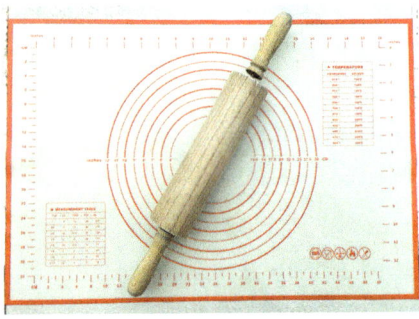

Silicone Rolling Mat

This is a great reusable and cost-effective mat to have in the kitchen. It provides a convenient non-stick work surface to work any of your doughs on. It's really easy to wash under the tap, and I've had mine for over five years now.

What to Use if You Don't Have a Silicone Rolling Mat
You can use cooking-liner sheets, which you can buy from most supermarkets or budget stores, or greaseproof paper.

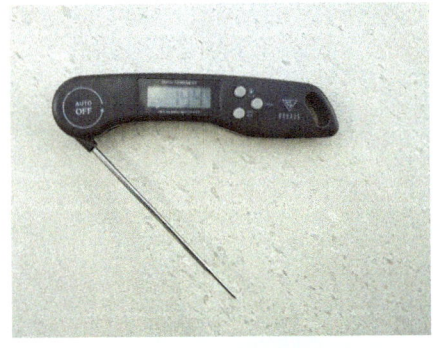

Kitchen Thermometer

Before I had a thermometer, I used to overcook everything, especially meat. Now, I would say, it's cooked to perfection. As for reheating meals, this also eliminates any cold spots.

I always make sure all meat and meals are 73°C or above.

What to Use if You Don't Have a Kitchen Thermometer
Unfortunately, there is no substitute, in my humble opinion.

Food
Is Your
Strength

You Are What You Eat

One Bolognese Four Ways

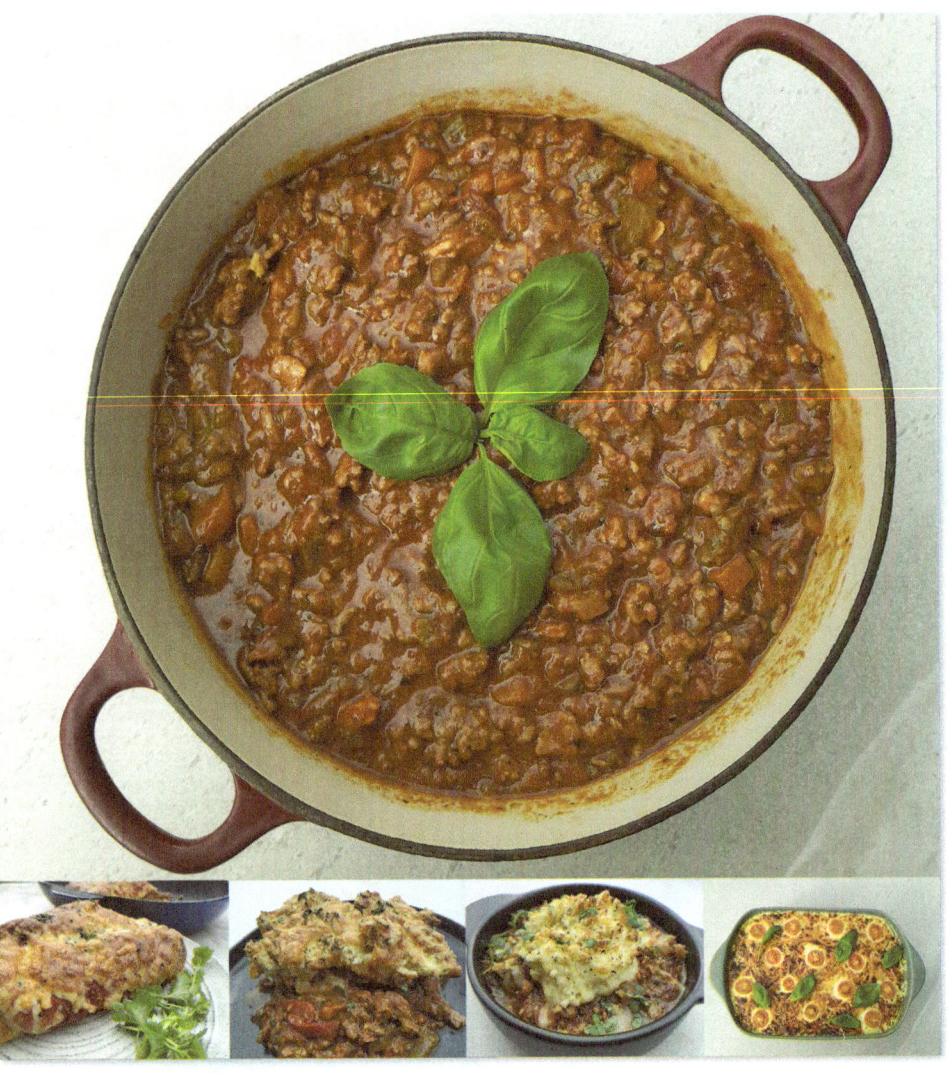

This is my base for so many mince-related dishes. My favourite is the baked enchiladas. I have a son who doesn't like red meat, so I swap the beef for chicken mince.

Equipment
- Large saucepan

Top Tips
- This can be frozen.

Making Time
Approximately 35–45 minutes

Makes
- 4 portions

Per Portion
- 8.7 g carbs / 30.7 g protein / 403 calories / 27.1g fat

Four Ways
Baked enchiladas (page 4); Chilli bake (page 6); Cottage pie (page 8); Lasagna (page 10).

INGREDIENTS
- 30g olive oil
- 75g bacon, chopped small
- 100g leeks, chopped small
- 50g carrots, chopped small
- 100g celery, chopped small
- 500g beef mince (or you could use, lamb, chicken or pork mince)
- 2 teaspoons garlic paste or 3 garlic cloves, finely chopped or crushed
- 1½ teaspoons oregano or mixed herbs
- 1 heaped teaspoon curry powder (not enough to taste it, but enough to give it an edge)
- 2 teaspoons paprika
- 1 tablespoon (15 g) tomato puree
- 400g tinned tomatoes (good quality)
- 200g boiling water to rinse out the tinned tomatoes and add to the pan
- 1 beef stock cube
- Salt and pepper (I add ½ teaspoon salt and ¼ teaspoon freshly ground black pepper)
- 10g 85% dark chocolate (this is included in the macros, but it is optional; it makes the meat sauce a lot richer, but you can't taste it)
- 15g basil to decorate

METHOD
1. Add the oil to a large non-stick saucepan and heat up until it's sizzling.
2. Add the chopped bacon, leeks, carrots and celery and cook for about 5 minutes until softened.
3. Add the meat, garlic and herbs to the saucepan. Carry on frying until the meat has browned, for about 5–10 minutes.
4. Add the curry powder, paprika and tomato puree and stir through.
5. Now add the tinned tomatoes.
6. Fill the empty tomato can with 200ml boiling water and dissolve the stock cube (this also helps to clean out the tomato tin) and add this to the saucepan and stir.
7. Season with the salt and pepper and stir through.
8. Now bring to a boil and simmer for at least 30 minutes, or until you're happy that the sauce has reduced to a beautiful thick bolognese. Add more water, if you need to.
9. Stir in the dark chocolate chunks until melted.
10. And, finally, top with basil leaves, or sprinkle on when serving. Enjoy! ♥

Baked Enchiladas

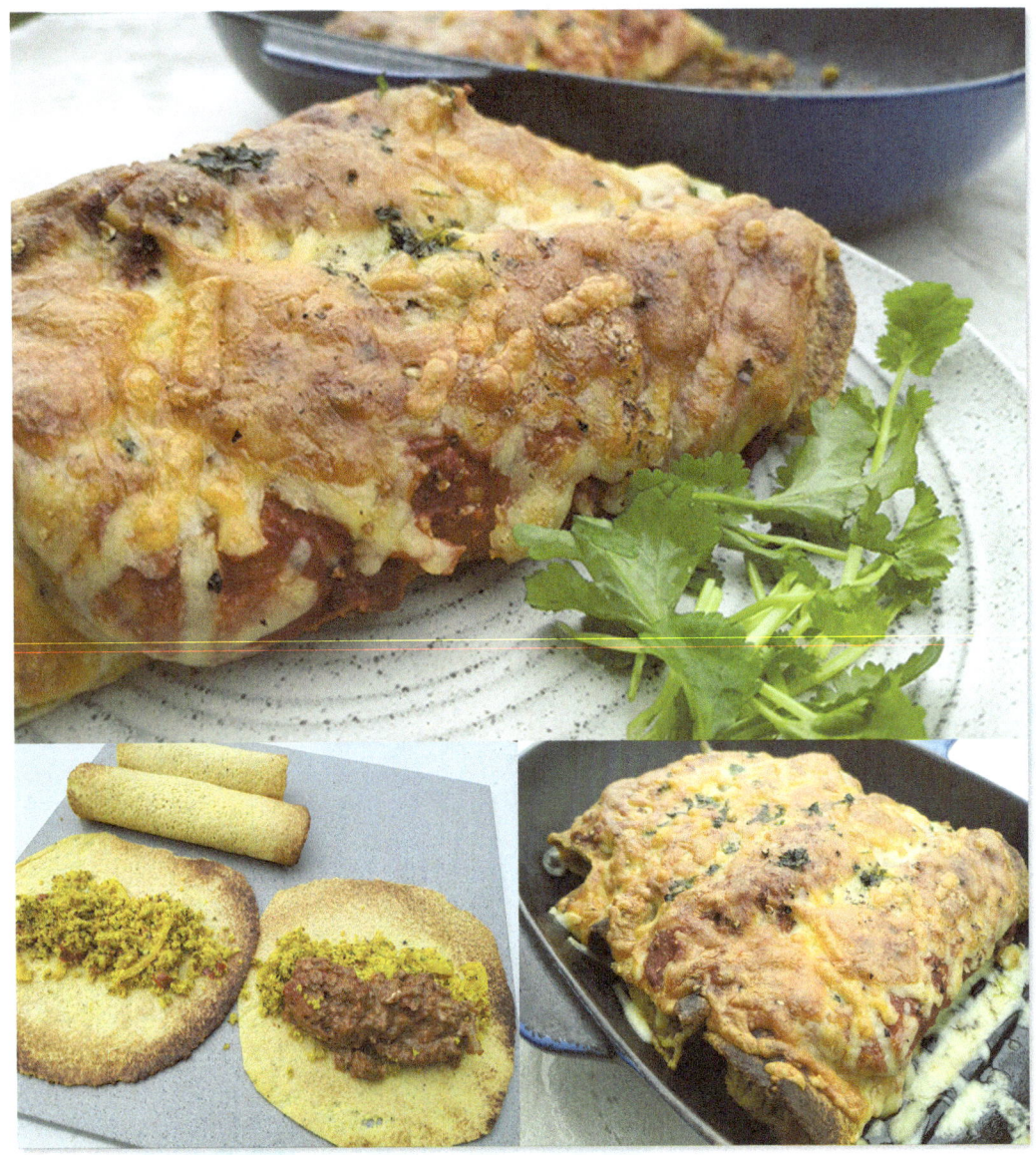

This is a cracking recipe, and to help make this a really easy recipe, I'd recommend using a tortilla press and a panini press (see pag xv for more information). They're not essential, but if you like wraps and pizzas, you'll love these two gadgets.

This is a fabulous meal to make in advance and just pop in the oven when you're ready. It can be eight starters for a nice Mexican meal, or four main-meal portions. It's super-filling and just wonderful.

You have a choice of two different wrap recipes: lupin wraps (page 96) and bamboo wraps (page 94). My favourite is lupin.

Equipment
- Large casserole dish (or several smaller ones)
- Greaseproof paper
- Rolling pin
- Food processor, bullet or hand blender
- Tortilla press (page xv)
- Panini flat-plate press (page xv)

Top Tips
- If you'd like to speed up the making time of this meal, omit the rice filling. It's what I do occasionally!
- If you're eating this later or defrosted and you would like to speed up the cooking process, heat it up in the microwave first then pop it under a hot grill for about 2 minutes to give it colour and a crispy cheese topping.
- This **can** be frozen.

Making Time
Approximately 45–50 minutes

Makes
8 enchiladas (4 portions: 2 enchiladas per person)

Per Portion
23.3g carbs / 59.2g protein / 884 calories / 58.9g fat (*including filling, using lupin wraps*)
19.9g carbs / 47.8g protein / 839 calories / 56.1g fat (*including filling, using bamboo wraps*)

INGREDIENTS

The Base Recipe
- 1 batch bolognese (page 2)
- 1 teaspoon Kashmiri chilli

The Wraps
- 8 of your chosen wrap recipe (for both the lupin wraps (page 96) and bamboo wraps (page 94), double the recipe)

The Rice Filling
- 30g butter
- 400g cauliflower, riced (blitz in a food processor until it resembles rice)
- ½ teaspoon turmeric
- Salt and pepper (I add ½ teaspoon salt and ¼ teaspoon freshly ground black pepper)
- 200g red peppers, chopped into fine strips

The Tomato Topping
- 400g tinned tomatoes (good quality)
- 2 ½ teaspoons paprika
- ½ teaspoon Kashmiri chilli powder (or your favourite chilli powder)
- ½ teaspoon garlic puree or 1 crushed garlic clove
- ½ teaspoon dried oregano or mixed herbs
- Salt and pepper (I add ½ teaspoon salt and ¼ teaspoon freshly ground black pepper)
- 1 teaspoon Truvia sweetener

And Finally
- 200g mature cheddar, grated

METHOD

The Base Recipe
1. Make the bolognese (page 2).
2. Add the Kashmiri chilli (1 teaspoon) to the bolognese while it's cooking.

The Wraps
3. While the bolognese is cooking, make up the wraps according to your chosen recipe.

The Rice Filling
4. Melt the butter in a non-stick frying pan. Add cauliflower rice, turmeric, seasoning and red-pepper strips.
5. Stir-fry until the cauliflower is cooked but not browned; this will take about 5–10 minutes.

The Tomato Topping
6. Add all the ingredients to a food processor, bullet or use a hand blender and blitz until smooth.

The Construction
7. Heat the oven to 180°C or the Ninja to 170°C.

Please refer to the pictures for guidance with this bit.

8. Have your wraps at the ready!
9. Divide your rice-and-pepper filling among the wraps.
10. Top with the bolognese shared between all the wraps.
11. Roll up the wraps and pop into an oven dish.
12. Pour the tomato topping over the top and sprinkle with cheese.
13. Cook for approx. 10 minutes or until it's piping hot in the middle. Enjoy! ♥

Chilli Bake

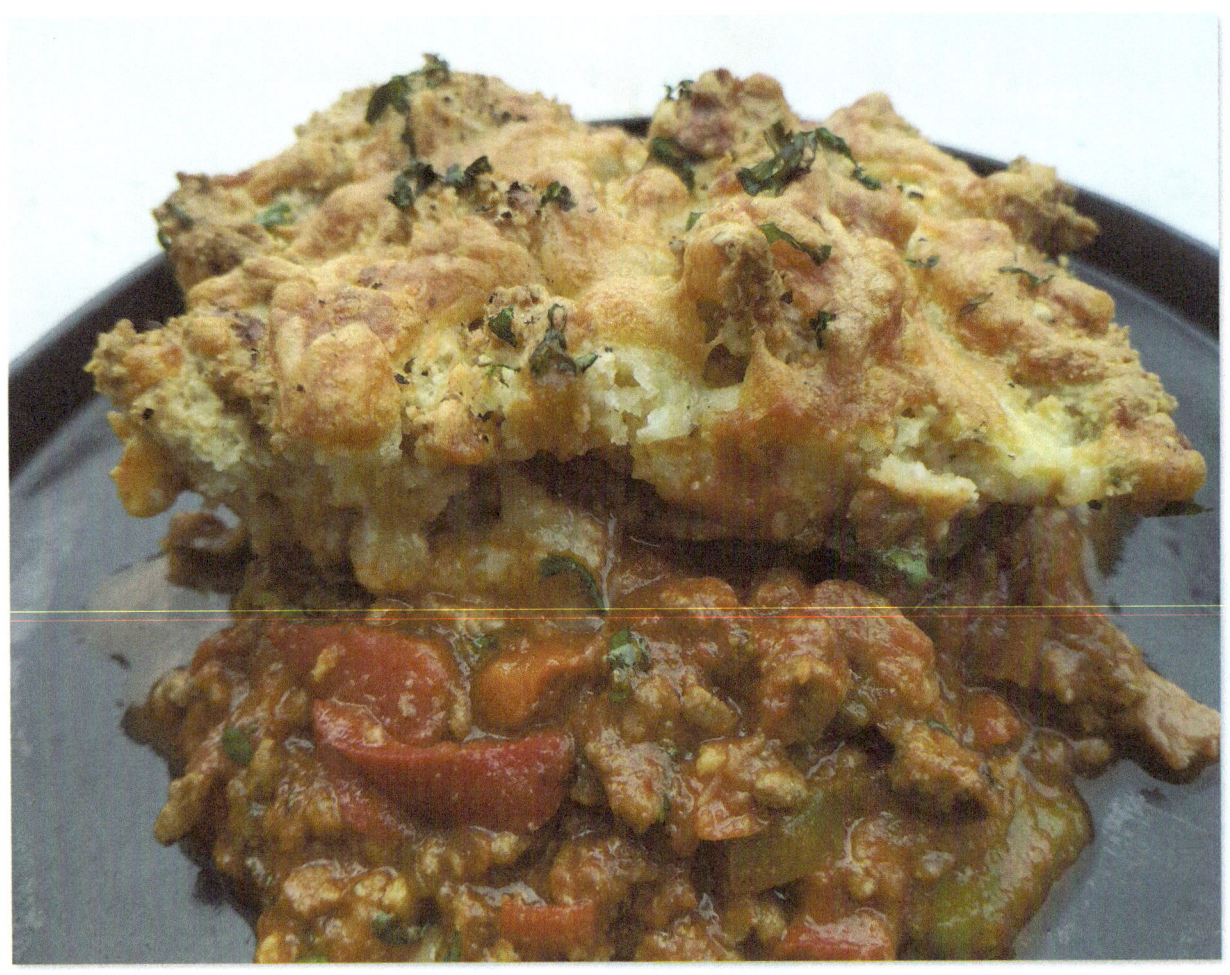

This is the sort of meal I like having as part of my OMAD (one meal a day) days. It's super filling just on its own and beautiful served with fresh salad. It's a spicy bolognese topped with a repurposed bread recipe, but, boy, does it work as a crispy topping. You'll love it!

Equipment
- Large non-stick saucepan
- Large mixing bowl
- Large casserole dish (or several smaller dishes for portion control)

Top Tips
- This **can** be frozen.
- If you'd like to speed this dish up, just omit 'The Chilli' section and add chilli, curry powder and coriander to the bolognese whilst it's cooking.

Making Time
Approximately 45–60 minutes

Makes
4 / 6 portions

Per Portion
15.5g carbs / 62.1g protein / 1095 calories / 85g fat (*if 4 portions*)
10.3g carbs / 41.4g protein / 730 calories / 56.7g fat (*if 6 portions*)

INGREDIENTS

The Base Recipe
- 1 batch bolognese (page 2)

The Chilli
- 250g red peppers (approx. 2 large, cored and deseeded), chunky chopped
- 10g olive oil
- 2 teaspoons curry powder
- 1 teaspoon Kashmiri chilli (this is to my taste; it has a nice bit of a kick, but it's a warm heat)
- 35g fresh coriander, finely chopped (keep a small bit back for decoration)

Optional Extra
- 100g borlotti beans (11.8g carbs/100 g — an extra 2.9g carbs per portion)

The Topping
- 130g ground almonds
- 130g milled golden linseed
- 10g psyllium husk
- 2 teaspoons baking powder
- Salt and pepper (I add ¼ teaspoon salt and ¼ teaspoon freshly ground black pepper)
- 150g mature cheddar, grated (save 50g for the topping)
- 100g cream cheese
- 4 eggs, medium

METHOD

The Base Recipe
1. Make the bolognese (page 2).
2. While the bolognese is cooking, move on to **Step 3** below.

The Chilli
3. Heat the oven to 200°C or the Ninja to 190°C.
4. Pop your peppers and olive oil into a baking tray and give them a good mix. Now bake for about 20–30 minutes until roasted (these can be fried in olive oil instead).
5. Add the rest of your chilli ingredients, including the roasted peppers, to the cooked bolognese base. Mix well, bring to temperature and gently simmer while you prepare the topping.
6. Add your beans now too, if you are using.

The Topping
7. Turn the oven down to 180°C or the Ninja to 170°C.
8. Add all the dry ingredients (including the cheddar, but hold back 50g of cheddar for topping) to a large bowl and mix.
9. Add all the wet ingredients to the dry mix, and mix well until you have a nice wet dough.
(Please note: the longer you leave this dough, the harder it is to spread.)

The Construction
10. Pour the chilli into a large casserole dish or 4/6 smaller casserole dishes.
11. Put small dollops of the bread dough across the top of the chilli then spread until even (the spreading isn't important—little chunky bits across the top are lovely too).
12. Sprinkle the final 50g grated cheddar all over the top and add a little freshly ground black pepper.
13. Bake for about 20–25 minutes until golden and cooked through. Enjoy! ♥

Cottage Pie

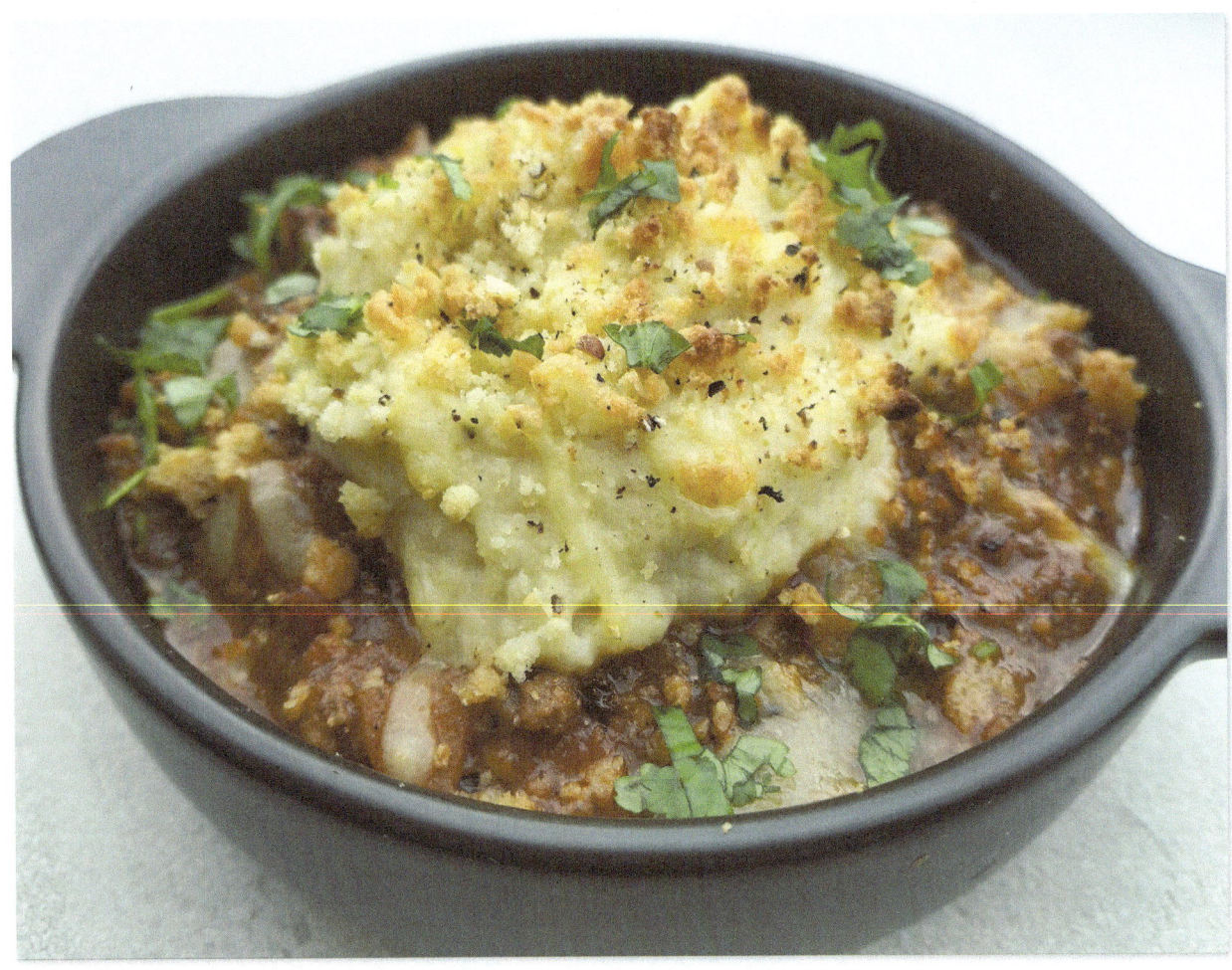

Good old comfort food. A lovely family dish with a beautiful crusty, cheesy topping. I've used a mix of cauliflower and swede for the mash topping, but there are lots of alternative low-carb vegetables that make a beautiful mash (page xiii). You'll love the mash.

Equipment
- Food processor or bullet
- Toaster
- Casserole dish (or 6 individual casserole dishes for portion control)
- Small microwave bowl for the bread

Top Tips
- This **can** be frozen.

Making Time
Approximately 60 minutes in total

Makes
4 / 6 portions

Per Portion
21.6g carbs / 43.3g protein / 621 calories / 40.5g fat (*if 4 portions*)
14.4g carbs / 28.8g protein / 414 calories / 27g fat (*if 6 portions*)

INGREDIENTS

The Base Recipe
- 1 batch bolognese (page 2)

The Mash Topping
- 450g cauliflower (including leaves), chunky chopped
- 450g swede, chunky chopped
- 50g cream cheese or double cream
- 50g mayonnaise (homemade (page 102) or your favourite shop-bought mayonnaise)
- Salt and pepper (I add ½ teaspoon salt and ¼ teaspoon freshly ground black pepper)

The Microwave Bread Topping (*this will make the breadcrumbs, or you could use your favourite low-carb bread—you'll need about 60g bread*).
- 35g ground almonds or ground seed or nut of your choice
- 1 medium egg
- ½ teaspoon baking powder
- Salt and pepper (I add ⅛ teaspoon salt and a good grind of black pepper)
- 50g mature cheddar cheese, grated (*add this at step 11*)

METHOD

The Base Recipe
1. Make the bolognese (page 2).
2. Heat oven to 190°C or the Ninja to 180°C.

The Mash Topping
3. Steam or boil your vegetables until they are totally and utterly soft, basically overcooked. (Trust me, this creates the perfect mash!)
4. Mash by hand, but even better if you have a food processor.
5. Add the cauliflower, swede, cream cheese, mayonnaise and seasoning to your food processor and mix until super smooth.

The Microwave Bread Topping
6. Mix all the ingredients apart from the cheese together in a microwaveable dish.
7. Microwave on full power for 90 seconds.
8. If you can, slice it and toast it. (This is to dry it out, so you can turn it into bread crumbs.)
9. Allow to cool slightly.
10. Whiz up in a food processor or Nutribullet until it resembles bread crumbs.
11. Mix in the grated cheddar.

The Construction
12. Pour the bolognese into a large casserole dish or 4/6 individual casserole dishes.
13. Put dollops of the mash across the top of the bolognese and then evenly spread across the top.
14. Sprinkle the cheesy bread crumbs over the mash.
15. Grind some black pepper over the top.
16. Bake for approximately 25–30 minutes. Enjoy! ♥

Lasagne

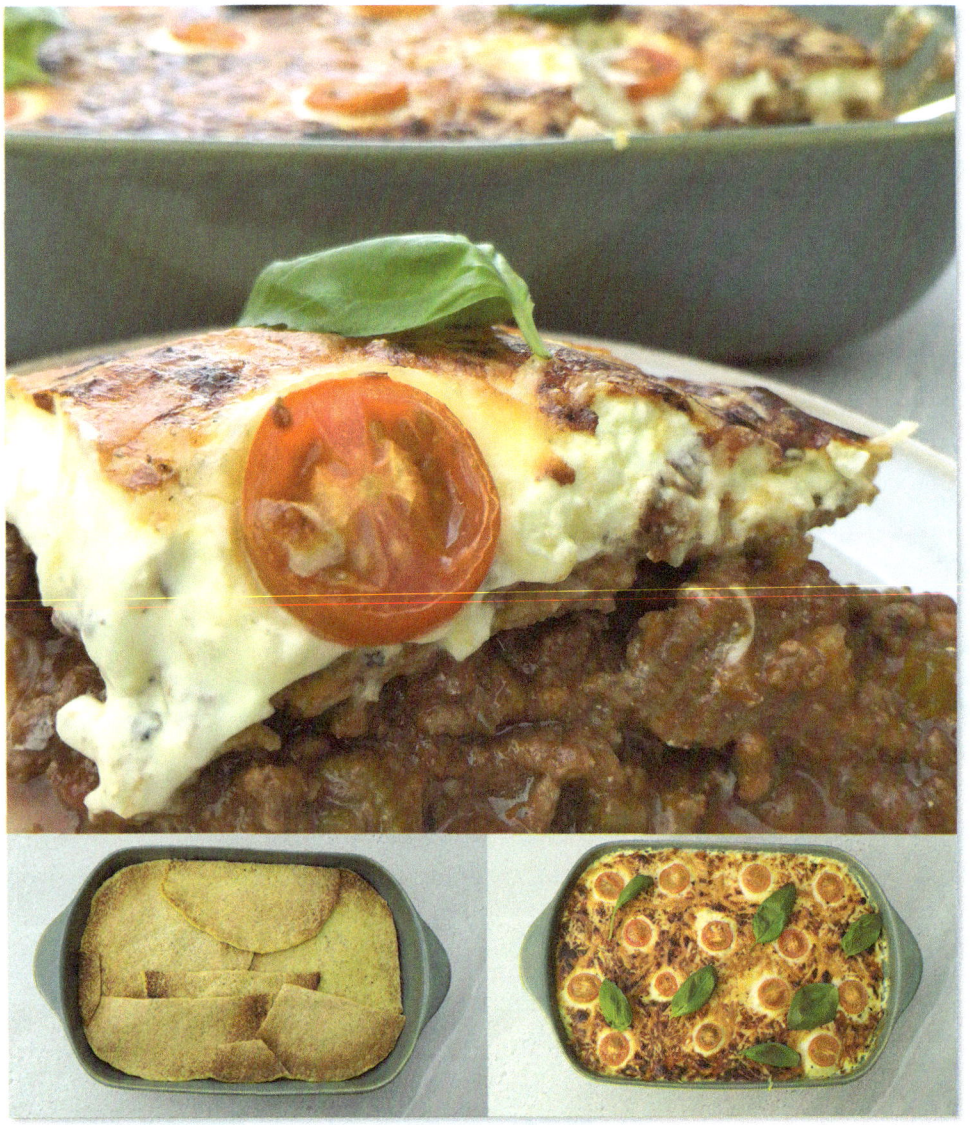

This is another fantastic family-pleaser meal. There are quite a few alternatives for the lasagne, so just choose your favourite lasagne sheet. My favourite is lupin wraps (page 96).

I'm going to give you three different lasagne alternatives for this recipe: bamboo wraps (page 94), lupin wraps (page 96) or MKD (Michele's keto dough) (page 98).

Equipment
- Lasagne dish (or 6 smaller casserole dishes)
- Large microwave bowl
- Greaseproof paper
- Rolling pin

Top Tips
- This **can** be frozen.

Making Time
Approximately 60 minutes

Makes
6 portions

Per Portion
10.3g carbs / 32.7g protein / 480 calories / 31.8g fat (*using bamboo wraps*)

11.4g carbs / 36.5g protein / 495 calories / 32.7g fat (*using lupin wraps*)

11.4g carbs / 42.1g protein / 610 calories / 43.2g fat (*using MKD*)

INGREDIENTS

The Base Recipe
- 1 batch bolognese (page 2)

Then choose your lasagne alternative, and follow those instructions.

The Wraps
- Bamboo wraps (page 94)
- Lupin wraps (page 96)
- MKD – Michele's Keto Dough (page 98)

The Rest of the Ingredients
- 400g crème fraiche
- 100g ready-grated mozzarella
- 1 teaspoon English mustard
- 50g parmesan, grated
- Salt and pepper (I add ½ teaspoon salt and ¼ teaspoon freshly grated black pepper)

The Toppings
- 10g basil
- 50g cherry tomatoes
- 50g mature cheddar cheese, grated

METHOD

The Base Recipe
1. Make the bolognese (page 2).

The Wraps
2. While the bolognese is cooking, make up your wraps according to your chosen wrap recipe: bamboo wraps (page 94), lupin wraps (page 96) or MKD (page 98).

The Sauce
3. In a bowl mix together the crème fraiche, mozzarella, English mustard, parmesan and seasoning.

The Construction
4. Heat oven to 190°C or the Ninja to 180°C.
5. Pour the bolognese into your lasagne dish.
6. Now pop your chosen wraps or cooked MKD sheet on top of the bolognese. Break it up or cut them to fit in the dish – refer to picture.
7. Pour the sauce over the top of the sheets and spread evenly.

The Toppings
8. Sprinkle with grated cheese and sliced cherry tomatoes to decorate.
9. Bake for approximately 30 minutes.
10. Once cooked, sprinkle lightly torn basil over the top. Enjoy! ♥

One Coleslaw
Four Ways

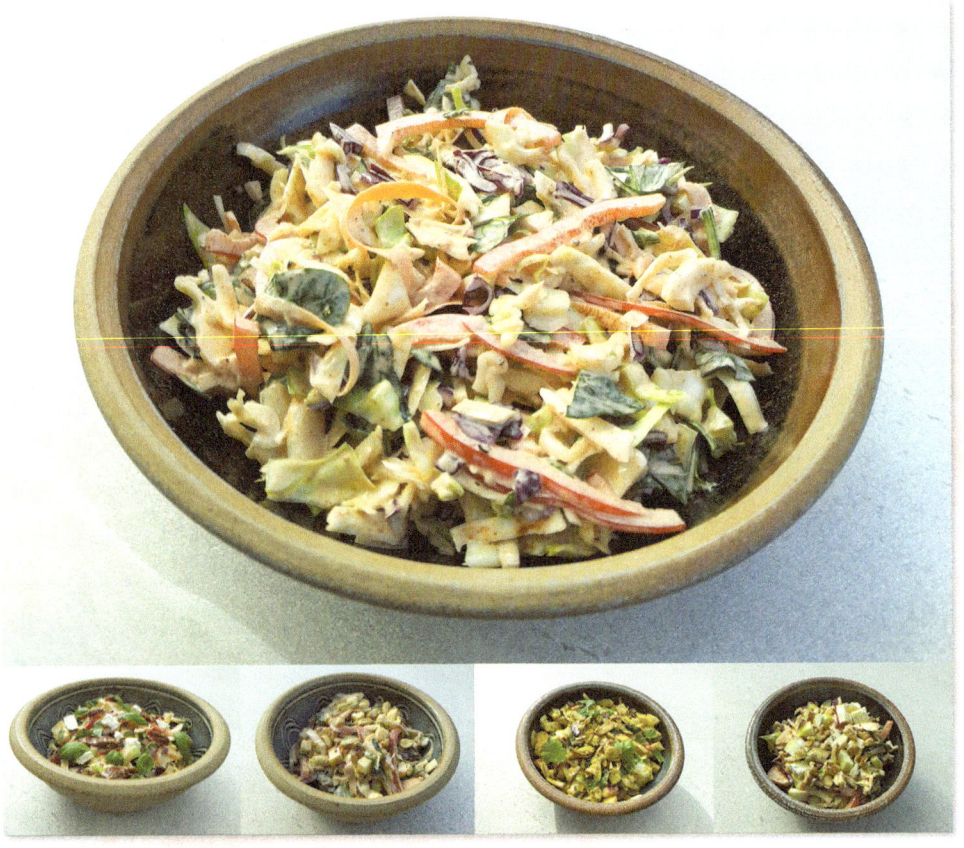

You can use just about any low carb vegetables that aren't predominantly soft, to make coleslaw. But in order to work out the macros, these are the ingredients that I love to use. So many combinations will work. The red pepper is in there for a touch of sweetness and the carrot and spinach are for extra colour, but not essential.

Equipment
- A sharp knife, or a food processor with the grating disc

Top Tips
- I choose **not** to freeze. Eat within approximately 3 days and keep in the fridge.
- If you have any coleslaw left over and are wondering what to do with it, it makes a fabulous stir fry.

Making Time
Approximately 10 minutes

Makes
4 portions

Per Portion
5g carbs / 2.4g protein / 211 calories / 20.2g fat

Four Ways
Basil, sundried tomatoes and feta (page 14); Cheddar and peanuts (pag15); Curried eggs (page 16); Stilton and walnut (page 17)

INGREDIENTS
- 225g white cabbage, finely chopped
- 60g red cabbage, finely chopped
- 60g sweetheart cabbage, finely chopped
- 75g red pepper, finely chopped
- 20g spinach, chunky chopped
- 10g carrot shavings (I like to add this for extra colour; use a potato peeler for this and take the skin off first)
- 100g homemade mayonnaise (page 102) or a mayonnaise of your choice
- 15g Will's chilli oil (page 106), or just add 1 tablespoon of olive oil and a pinch of chilli powder
- Salt and pepper (I add ½ teaspoon salt and ¼ teaspoon of freshly ground pepper)

METHOD
1. If you are using homemade mayonnaise, you'll need to make this first (page 102).
2. Once prepared, add all your ingredients to a large bowl and mix. Enjoy! ♥

Basil, Sundried Tomatoes and Feta

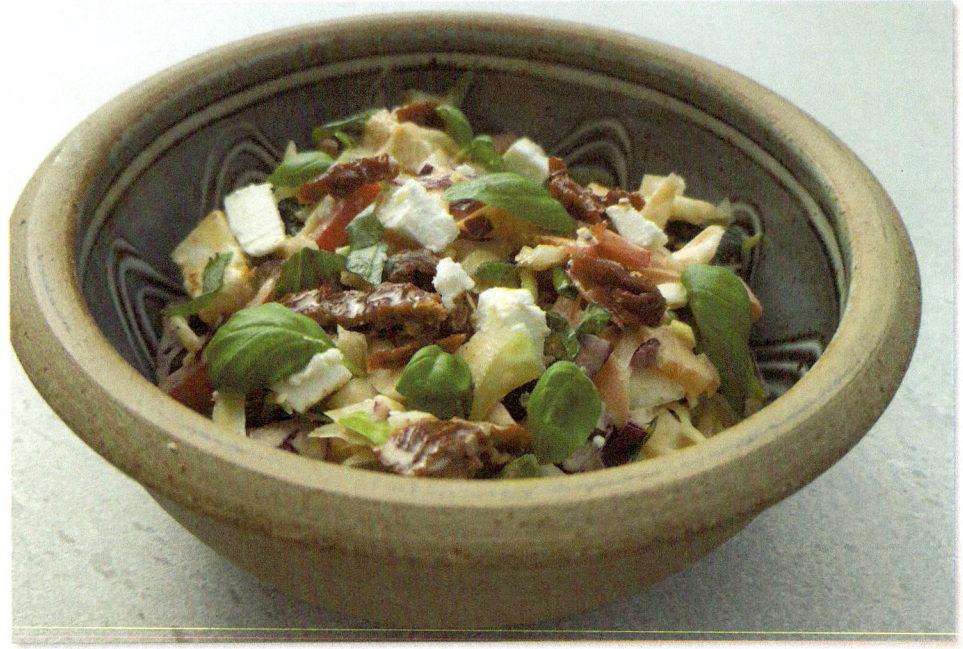

Once you've made the base recipe, you just add the three ingredients from the list below. Easy.

Equipment
- A sharp knife, or a food processor with the grating disc

Top Tips
- I choose **not** to freeze. Eat within approximately 3 days and keep in the fridge.
- If you have any coleslaw left over, it makes a fabulous stir-fry.

Making Time
Approximately 12 minutes

Makes
4 portions

Per Portion
6.3g carbs / 5.9g protein / 293 calories / 26.8g fat

INGREDIENTS
The Base Recipe
- 1 batch coleslaw (page 12)

The Rest of the Ingredients
75g sundried tomatoes, chunky chopped
75g feta, chopped into small cubes
20g basil, lightly torn up into small pieces or chunky chopped with a knife

METHOD
The Base Recipe
1. Make the coleslaw (page 12)

Now the Final Parts of the Recipe
2. Add the sundried tomatoes, cubed feta and basil to the coleslaw and stir through. Enjoy! ♥

Cheddar and Peanuts

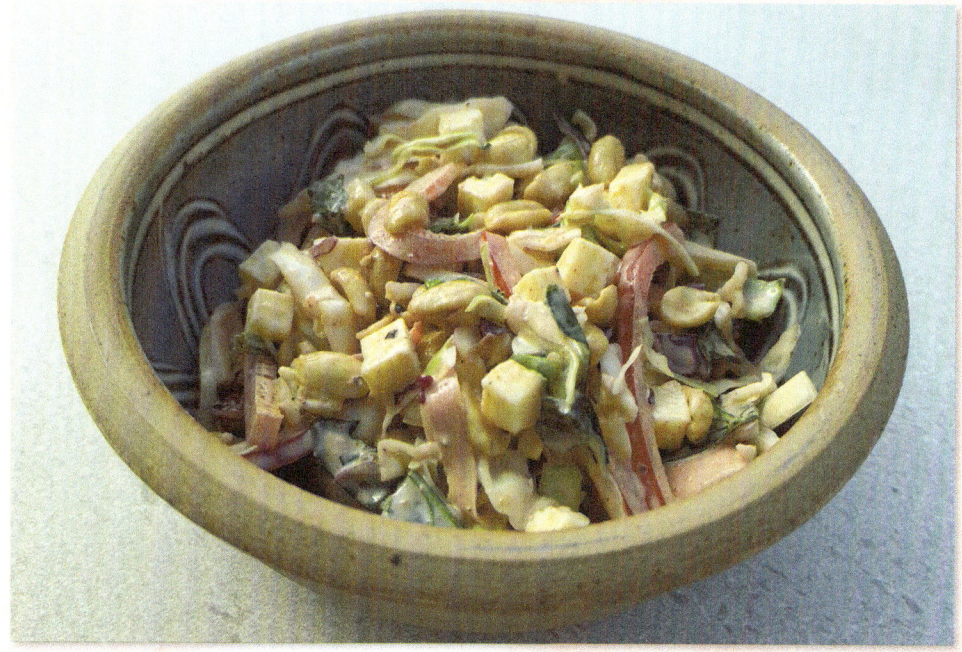

Once you've made the base recipe, you just add the two ingredients from the list below. If I'm making this to take to friends or family for dinner, I add the peanuts just before I set off. At home I add immediately and accept that the peanuts will soften slightly.

Equipment
- A sharp knife, or a food processor with the grating disc

Top Tips
- If you want maximum crunch in the peanuts, add them just before serving; however, it does not take away from the taste of this dish if you decide to add them straightaway.
- I choose **not** to freeze. Eat within approximately 3 days and keep in the fridge.
- If you have any coleslaw left over, it makes a fabulous stir-fry.

Making Time
Approximately 12 minutes

Makes 4 portions

Per Portion
6.4g carbs / 11.8g protein / 402 calories / 36.7g fat

INGREDIENTS

The Base Recipe
- 1 batch coleslaw (page 12)

The Rest of the Ingredients
- 75g mature cheddar, chopped into small cubes about 1 cm square
- 75g peanuts (I prefer salted peanuts)

METHOD

The Base Recipe
1. Make the coleslaw (page 12)

Now the Final Parts of the Recipe
2. Add the cubed cheddar and peanuts to the base and stir through. Enjoy! ♥

Curried Eggs

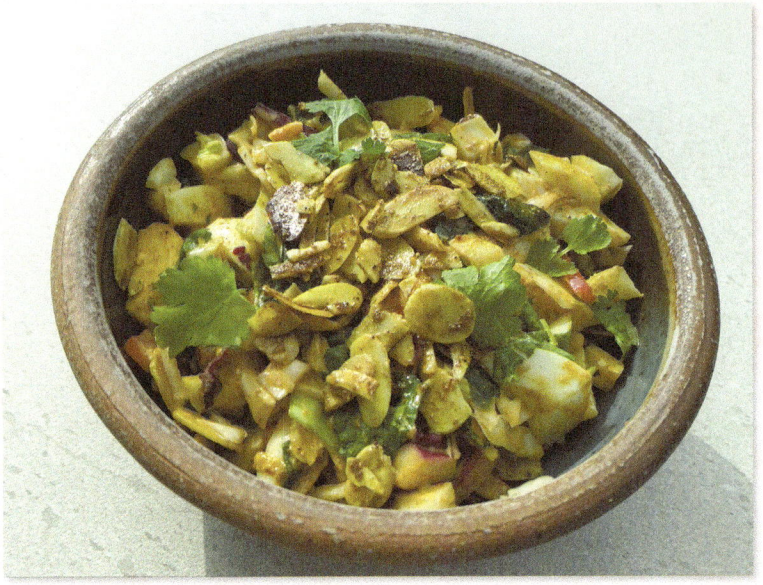

Once you've made the base recipe, you just add a little taste of magic to the boiled eggs and then add a few extra ingredients from the list below.

Equipment
- A sharp knife, or a food processor with the grating disc
- Non-stick frying pan

Top Tips
- This **cannot** be frozen. Eat within approximately 3 days and keep in the fridge.
- If you have any coleslaw left over, it makes a fabulous stir-fry.

Making Time
Approximately 15 minutes

Makes
4 portions

Per Portion
5.9g carbs / 10.8g protein / 388 calories / 35.8g fat

INGREDIENTS

The Base Recipe
- 1 batch coleslaw (page 12)

The Rest of the Ingredients
- 30g olive oil
- 4 hard-boiled eggs, peeled but left whole
- 30g flaked almonds
- 6 teaspoons curry powder
- 4 tablespoons fresh coriander, roughly chopped

METHOD

The Base Recipe
1. Make the coleslaw (page 12)

Now the Final Parts of the Recipe
2. Add oil to the pan and heat up until sizzling, then add the curry powder and stir.
3. Add the whole hard-boiled eggs and flaked almonds to the pan.
4. Fry for about 2 minutes, stirring occasionally.
5. Allow to cool.
6. Once cool, chunky chop the egg.
7. Now add the eggs, flaked almonds, pan juices and fresh coriander to the base and stir through. Enjoy! ♥

Stilton and Walnut, and Optional Apple

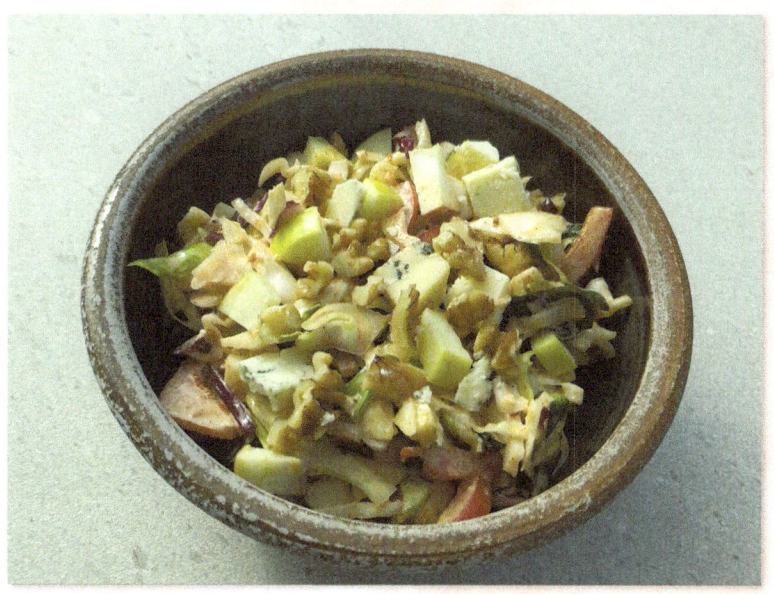

Once you've made the base recipe, you just add the two (or three if you're adding apple as well) ingredients, from the list below.

Equipment
- A sharp knife, or a food processor with the grating disc.

Making Time
Approximately 12 minutes

Makes
4 portions

Per Portion
5.5g carbs / 8.4g protein / 369 calories / 34.9g fat

Top Tips
- If you want maximum crunch in the walnuts, add them just before serving; however, it does not take away from the taste of this dish if you decide to add them straightaway.
- I choose **not** to freeze. Eat within approximately 3 days and keep in the fridge.
- If you have any coleslaw left over, it makes a fabulous stir-fry.

INGREDIENTS

The Base Recipe
- 1 batch coleslaw (page 12)

The Rest of the Ingredients
- 50g walnuts, chunky chopped
- 70g Stilton (this will be crumbled in with your fingers at the end)

Optional Extra (this will increase the carbs, but it adds a lovely sweetness)
- 50g apple (approximately 1 small eating apple), chunky chopped (with skin if it's an eating apple, and without the skin if it's a cooking apple). For a Granny Smith apple, add 2.9g carbs per portion and for a Bramley cooking apple add 2.2g carbs per portion.

METHOD

The Base Recipe
1. Make the coleslaw (page 12)

Now the Final Parts of the Recipe
2. Dry fry the walnuts in a non-stick pan for about 2 minutes, to give them a lovely roasted flavour, then allow to cool.
3. Add the fried walnuts to the coleslaw base and crumble in the Stilton with your fingertips. Then add the apple if you choose to and stir through. Enjoy! ♥

One Crustless Quiche
Four Ways

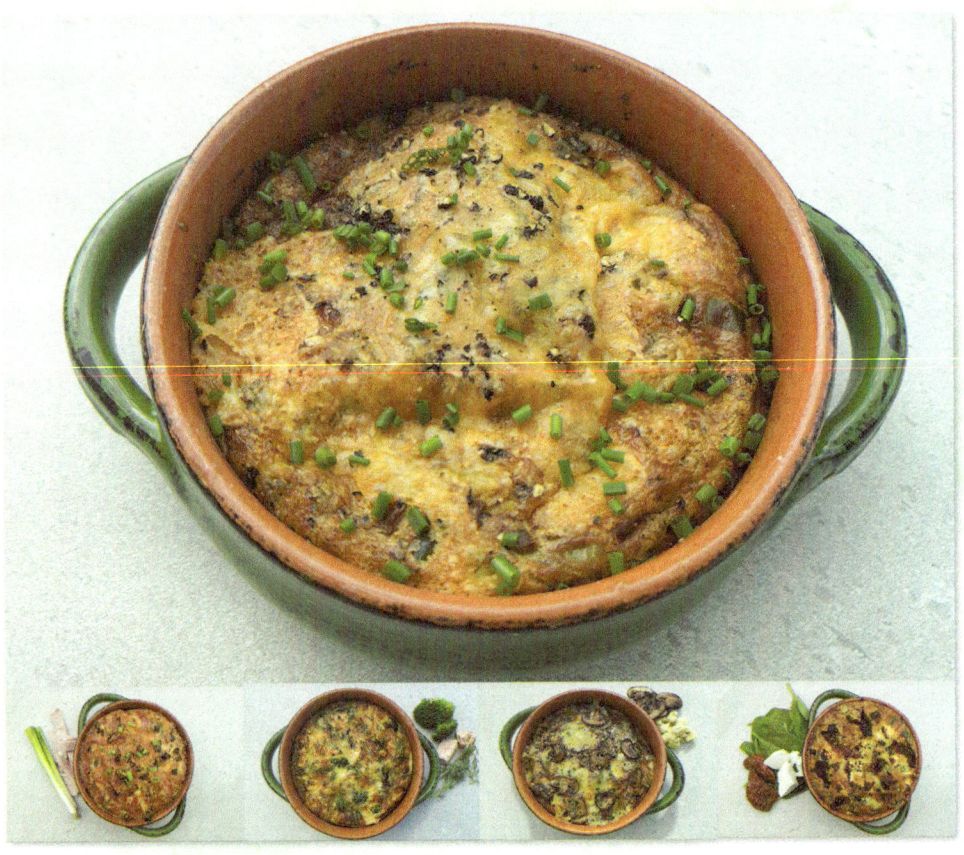

I spent a long time researching the perfect pastry, and there are some great low-carb recipes out there. I've also used corned-beef slices, which works really well too. However, what I particularly like about these recipes is their simplicity, yet still with all the flavour, and so much quicker and easier to make without the pastry crust.

If you would like a crust, I have two fabulous alternative pastry recipes to choose from: the pie crust (page 32) or the standard pastry recipe used in the custard tart (page 82).

If you cook this as a tray bake in a brownie tin, it makes great party food. You could get as many as 15 portions.

Equipment
- Non-stick saucepan
- Large mixing bowl
- A lined or well-greased shallow ovenproof dish. If you are using the Ninja grill, just line it with a silicone sheet.

Top Tips
- If you'd like to reduce the fat and calories, you could half the cream and replace it with your favourite milk. I like to use full-fat lactose-free milk.
- Allow to cool completely before slicing.
- This **can** be frozen.

Four Ways
Ham and spring onion (page 20); Salmon and broccoli (page 21); Stilton and mushroom (page 22) Sundried tomatoes, spinach and feta (page 23)

Making Time Approximately 45 minutes

Makes 4 / 6 portions

Per Portion
3.5g carbs / 22g protein / 749 calories / 71.8g fat (*if 4 portions*)
2.3g carbs / 14.7g protein / 499 calories / 47.9g fat (*if 6 portions*)

INGREDIENTS
- 20g butter
- 20g olive oil
- 150g leeks, thinly sliced
- ½ teaspoon garlic paste or 1 garlic clove crushed or finely chopped
- 6 medium eggs
- 300ml double cream
- 100g cream cheese
- Salt and pepper (I add ½ teaspoon salt and ¼ teaspoon freshly ground pepper)
- 150g grated cheddar (**hold back 50g for the topping**)

METHOD
1. Heat the oven to 180°C or the Ninja to 160°C.
2. Grease or line your baking dish (as long as it's ovenproof, anything works).
3. In a non-stick frying pan, add the butter and oil and heat until the butter has melted.
4. Add the leeks and cook for about 5 minutes, until the leeks are cooked but not browned. *If you're making the Stilton and mushroom quiche, add the mushrooms now too.*
5. Stir through the garlic and cook for a further minute, then allow to cool slightly before adding to the egg mix (below).
6. Meanwhile, in a large bowl, whisk up the eggs, cream, cream cheese, seasoning and mix well. Using a fork is absolutely fine.
7. Add the cooled leeks and grated cheese (**hold some cheese back for the topping**) and stir through.
8. **If you are now making any of the following quiches, stop here and finish off within the recipe of your choice:**
   - Ham and spring onion (page 20)
   - Salmon and broccoli (page 21)
   - Stilton and mushroom (page 22)
   - Sundried tomatoes, feta and spinach (page 23)

Back to the Base
9. Pour the egg mix into your greased ovenproof dish.
10. Bake for about 30–45 minutes, or until it's not wobbly.
11. This will rise then shrink back a little. Enjoy! ♥

Ham and Spring Onion

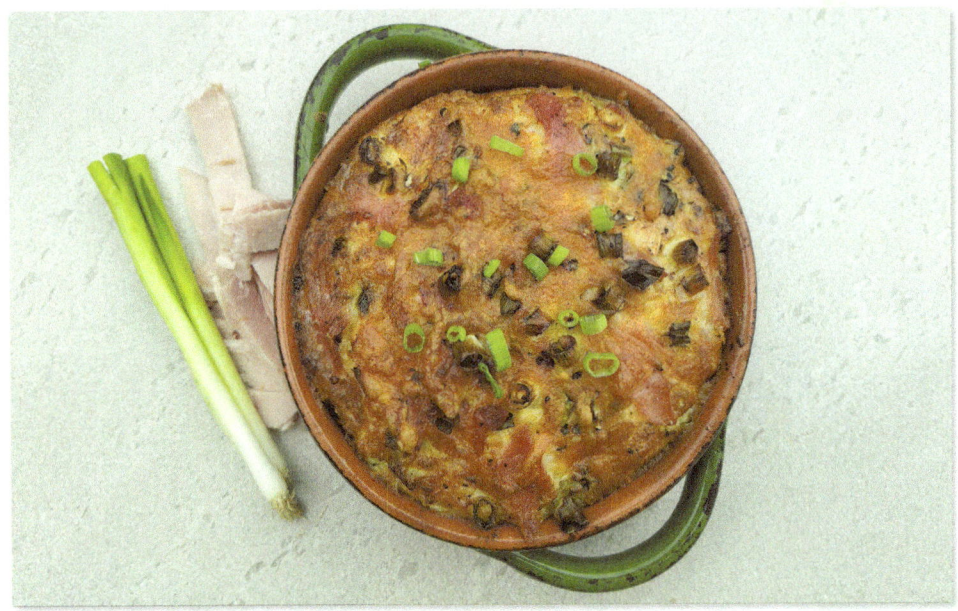

This is the quickest quiche of the four recipes and is so delicious

Equipment
- Non-stick saucepan
- Large mixing bowl
- Ovenproof dish, refer to base for details (page 18)

Top Tips
- Allow to cool completely before slicing.
- This **can** be frozen.

Making Time Approximately 45 minutes

Makes 4 / 6 portions

Per Portion
4.3g carbs / 36g protein / 841 calories / 74.9g fat
(*if 4 portions*)
2.9g carbs / 24g protein / 561 calories / 50g fat
(*if 6 portions*)

INGREDIENTS

The Base Recipe
- 1 batch crustless quiche (page 18)

The Rest of the Ingredients
- 250g cooked gammon or your favourite ham, chunky chopped
- 50g spring onion, finely sliced

METHOD

The Base Recipe
1. Make the crustless quiche (page 18). Stop after you have done **Step 7** and come back to this recipe.

Now the Final Parts of the Recipe
2. Add the gammon and spring onion to the egg mix and stir through (hold back a little of the gammon and spring onion to decorate the top of the quiche).
3. Pour the mixture into your prepared oven dish and decorate with your leftover gammon and spring onion and the final bit of grated cheese.
4. Bake for about 30–45 minutes, or until it's not wobbly.
5. This will rise then shrink back a little. Enjoy! ♥

Salmon, Broccoli and Dill

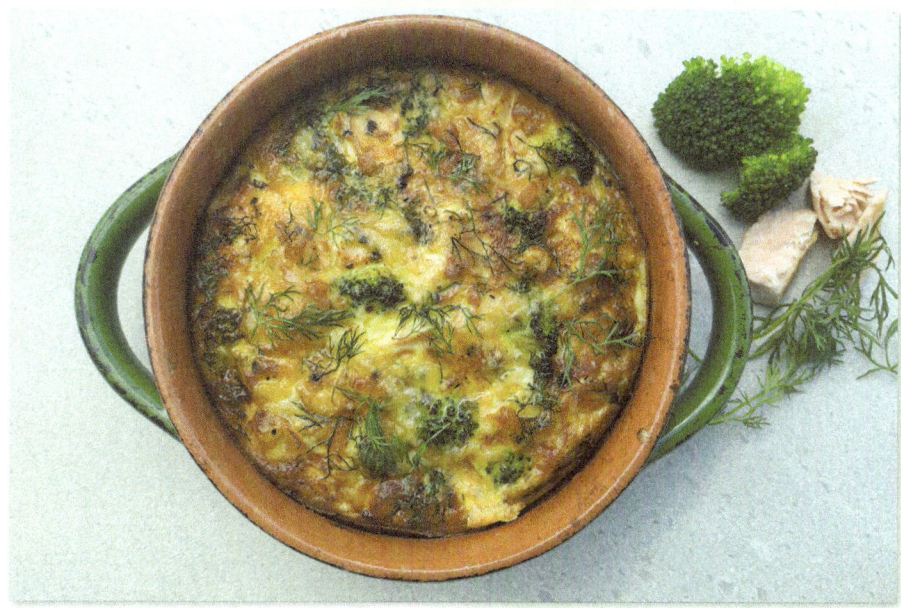

This will work with most fish. Occasionally, I swap it for a small amount of anchovies.

Equipment
- Non-stick saucepan
- Large mixing bowl
- Ovenproof dish, refer to base for details (page 18)

Top Tips
- Allow to cool completely before slicing.
- This **can** be frozen.

Making Time Approximately 45 minutes

Makes 4 / 6 portions

Per Portion
4.3g carbs / 35.9g protein / 893 calories / 81.3g fat (*if 4 portions*)
2.9g carbs / 23.9g protein / 596 calories / 54.2g fat (*if 6 portions*)

INGREDIENTS

The Base Recipe
- 1 batch crustless quiche (page 18)

The Rest of the Ingredients
- 250g fresh salmon (if you prefer, you could use smoked salmon for a more smoky taste
- 100g broccoli, chunky chopped
- 1 tablespoon fresh dill, chopped up small

METHOD

The Salmon & Broccoli
1. Firstly, you'll need to cook the salmon. The salmon can be grilled, baked or steamed. If you are using smoked salmon, there's nothing to do apart from break it up into chunks.
2. Steam or boil your broccoli. Try not to over cook it, then immediately transfer it to cold water. This helps to retain its colour and then drain.

The Base Recipe
3. Make the crustless quiche (page 18). Stop after you have done **Step 7** and come back to this recipe.

Now the Final Parts of the Recipe
4. Add the cooked salmon, broccoli and dill to the egg mix and stir through (*hold back a little of the salmon, broccoli and dill to decorate the top of the quiche*).
5. Pour the mixture into your prepared oven dish and decorate with your leftover salmon, broccoli and dill and the final bit of grated cheese.
6. Bake for about 30–45 minutes, or until it's not wobbly.
7. This will rise then shrink back a little. Enjoy! ♥

Stilton and Mushroom

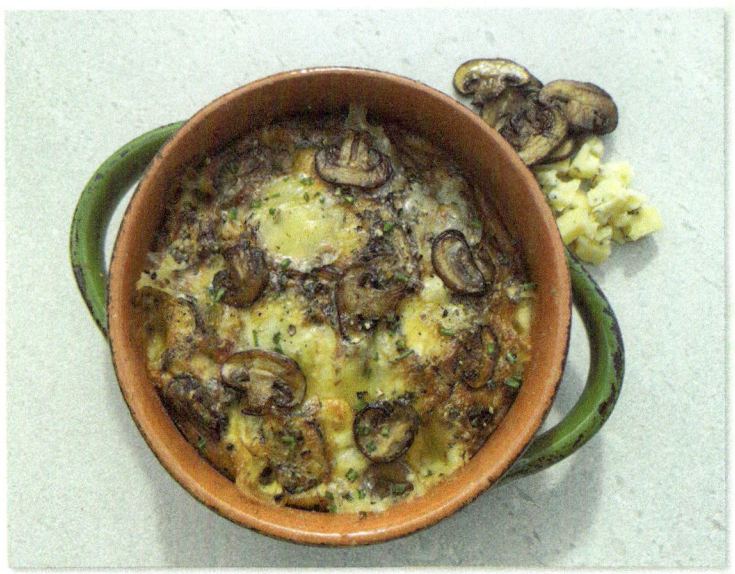

This is my absolute favourite of the quiches. It's so rich and gooey, with a really punchy flavour.

Equipment
- Non-stick saucepan
- Large mixing bowl
- Ovenproof dish, refer to base for details (page 18)

Top Tips
- Allow to cool completely before slicing.
- This **can** be frozen.

Making Time Approximately 45 minutes

Makes 4 / 6 portions

Per Portion
3.7g carbs / 28.5g protein / 856 calories / 80.7g fat (*if 4 portions*)
2.5g carbs / 19g protein / 570 calories / 53.8g fat (*if 6 portions*)

INGREDIENTS

The Base Recipe
- 1 batch crustless quiche (page 18)

The Rest of the Ingredients
- 200 g mushrooms, chunky chopped, or sliced (I prefer to use chestnut mushrooms, as I love the texture and taste of them, but any mushrooms will work)
- 100 g Stilton, lightly crumbled with your fingers

METHOD

The Base Recipe
1. Make crustless quiche (page 18).
2. Add the mushrooms at **Step 4** of the base recipe and carry on until you've completed **Step 7**.

Now the Final Parts of the Recipe
3. Add the Stilton to the egg mixture and stir through (*hold back a little of the Stilton to decorate the top of the quiche*).
4. Pour the mixture into your prepared oven dish and decorate with your leftover Stilton and the final bit of grated cheese.
5. Bake for about 30–45 minutes, or until it's not wobbly.
6. This will rise then shrink back a little. Enjoy! ♥

Sundried Tomatoes, Spinach and Feta

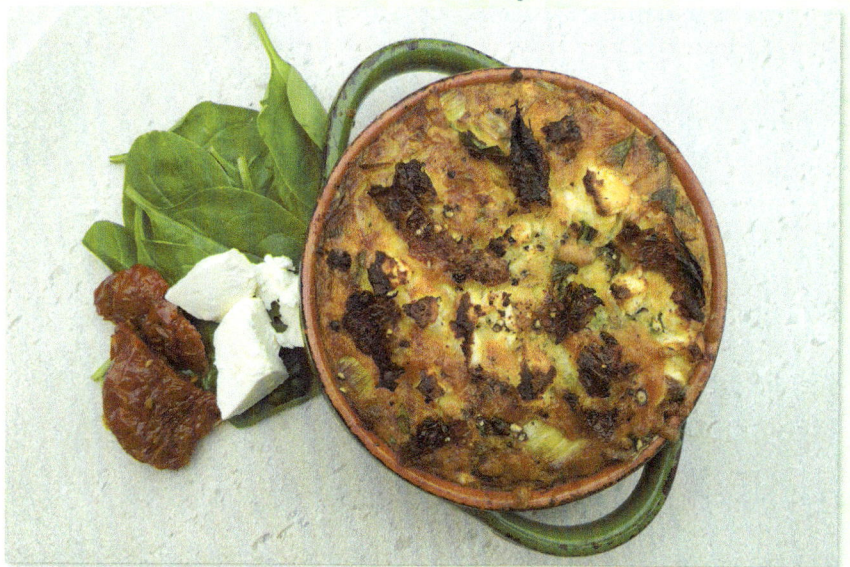

When you slice into this quiche, you see it has the most incredible layers, which look absolutely beautiful. The taste is great too.

Equipment
- Non-stick saucepan
- Large mixing bowl
- Ovenproof dish, refer to base for details (page 18)

Top Tips
- Allow to cool completely before slicing.
- This **can** be frozen.

Making Time Approximately 45 minutes

Makes
4 / 6 portions

Per Portion
5.1g carbs / 26.8g protein / 858 calories / 80.7g fat (*if 4 portions*)
3.4g carbs / 17.9g protein / 572 calories / 53.8g fat (*if 6 portions*)

INGREDIENTS

The Base Recipe
- 1 batch crustless quiche (page 18)

The Rest of the Ingredients
- 50g spinach, chunky chopped
- 100g sundried tomatoes, finely chopped (go for the lowest carb you can find — mine was 4 g/100 g)
- 100g feta, crumbled with your fingers

METHOD

The Base Recipe
1. Make the crustless quiche (page 18). Stop after you have done **Step 7** and come back to this recipe.

Now the Final Parts of the Recipe
2. Add the spinach, sundried tomatoes and feta to the egg mix and stir through (*hold back a little of the sundried tomatoes, spinach and feta to decorate the top of the quiche*).
3. Pour the mix into your prepared oven dish and decorate with your leftover sundried tomatoes and feta and the final bit of grated cheese.
4. Bake for about 30–45 minutes, or until it's not wobbly.
5. This will rise then shrink back a little. Enjoy! ♥

One Curry
Four Ways

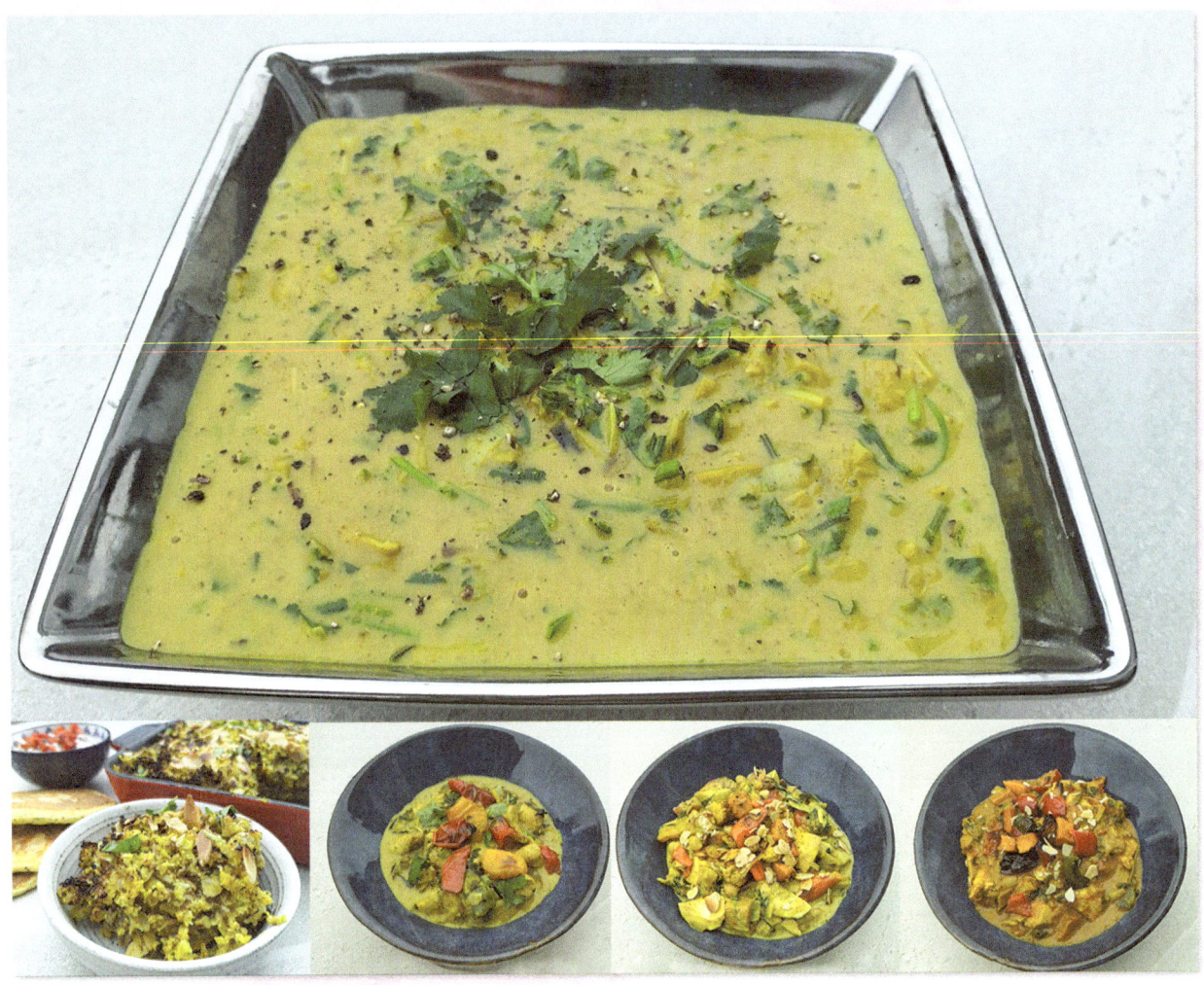

This makes a fab sauce on its own. Just pour it over your cooked protein, or add king prawns, boiled eggs or dry-fried halloumi. Beautiful.

Equipment
- Large saucepan

Top Tips
- I'm a big fan of fresh coriander, so you don't have to use as much as I have in the recipe. If you don't like coriander, swap it for spinach, which has a similar wilting texture. When I haven't had either in the house, I've also swapped it for curly kale.
- This **can** be frozen.

Making Time
Approximately 20 minutes

Makes
4 portions

Per Portion
6.7g carbs / 2.5g protein / 264 calories / 25.5g fat

Four Ways
Biryani (page 26); Chicken and roast pepper curry (page 28); Roasted vegetable and butter bean curry (page 29); Chicken, tomato and roasted vegetable curry (page 30)

INGREDIENTS
- 40g butter or coconut oil
- 200g leeks, chunky chopped
- 2 teaspoons garlic puree or 3 garlic cloves, finely chopped
- 2 teaspoons ginger puree or 2½ teaspoons fresh ginger, chopped finely
- 6 teaspoons curry powder
- 400g coconut milk, tinned (the highest percentage of coconut extract you can find)
- 30g fresh coriander, finely chopped
- 15ml freshly squeezed lime or lemon juice
- Salt and pepper (I use ½ teaspoon salt and ¼ teaspoon freshly ground black pepper)

METHOD
1. Add the butter or oil to a large non-stick pan and heat up until sizzling.
2. Turn down to a medium heat and add the leeks and fry for about 5 minutes or until the leeks start to go translucent, but not brown, and are cooked.
3. Add the garlic and ginger and stir through and fry for 1 minute.
4. Now add the curry powder and stir through and fry for a further minute.
5. Add the coconut milk and allow it to come back to almost boiling, then turn it down to a gentle simmer for about 5 minutes.
6. Add the coriander, lime juice, seasoning and stir.
7. Your curry base is complete. You can now choose which recipe you'd like to make, or just use it as a lovely sauce with a protein of your choice. Enjoy! ♥

Biryani

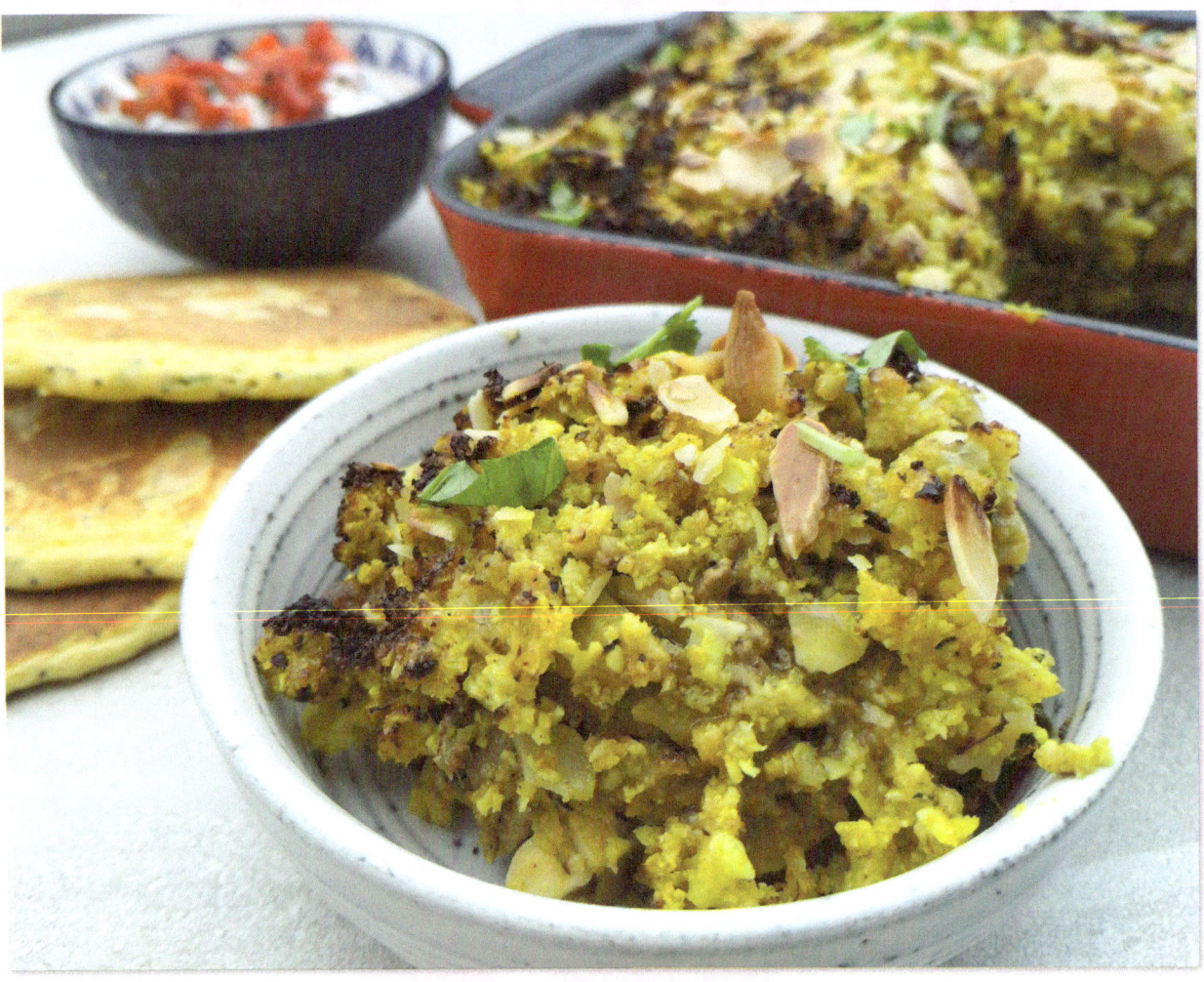

This is my absolute favourite of the curries. But it is also the curry that I make the least because it is more time consuming than the others. But if you have the time it does not disappoint.

Equipment
- 2 large non-stick pans
- Food processor, for ricing the vegetables
- Large ovenproof dish

Top Tips
- This **can** be frozen.

Making Time
Approximately 60 minutes

Makes
4 portions

Per Portion
17.3g carbs / 34.8g protein / 700 calories / 54.8g fat

INGREDIENTS

The Base Recipe
- 1 batch curry (page 24)

The Rest of the Ingredients
- 700g fresh cauliflower, whizzed up in the food processor to resemble rice
- ½ teaspoon ground turmeric
- Seasoning for the cauliflower (I add ½ teaspoon salt and ¼ teaspoon freshly ground pepper)
- 40g butter (20g for frying the cauliflower, 5g to grease the casserole dish and 15g to dot on top of the finished dish)
- 500g beef/lamb mince
- 1 teaspoon curry powder
- Seasoning for the mince (I add ¼ teaspoon salt and ¼ teaspoon freshly ground pepper)
- 200g tinned tomatoes (good quality)
- 40g flaked almonds

Optional Extras
- Greek yogurt or sour cream as a garnish
- Extra coriander to decorate

METHOD

The Base Recipe
1. Make the curry (page 24).

The Rest of the Recipe

2. Meanwhile, mix the ground turmeric and salt and pepper into the riced-up cauliflower.
3. Melt the butter (20g) in a large non-stick frying pan and then add the seasoned cauliflower. Stir regularly, lifting the cauliflower so it's completely cooked. This will take about 10 minutes. Put to one side.
4. In another large non-stick pan add the mince and fry off until crispy (approximately 10 minutes).
5. To the mince add the curry powder, salt and pepper. Mix well and fry for a further minute.
6. Now add the tinned tomatoes and cooked mince to your prepared curry base recipe and stir well.

Biriyani Construction

7. Heat the oven to 190°C or the Ninja to 180°C.
8. Grease a large casserole dish with 5g butter. **You're now going to do your layers.**
9. **Layer 1:** Put a third of the cauliflower in the base of the greased dish and spread out evenly.
10. **Layer 2:** Add half of the curry over the cauliflower and spread evenly.
11. **Layer 3:** Put the next third of the cauliflower on top of the curry layer and spread out evenly.
12. **Layer 4:** Evenly spread the other half of the curry over the cauliflower.
13. **Layer 5:** Put the final third of the cauliflower on top of the curry layer and spread out evenly.
14. Sprinkle flaked almonds over the top of the cauliflower rice.
15. Dot with the remaining 15g butter and season with freshly ground black pepper.
16. Loosely cover with foil and cook for approximately 30–40 minutes, or until completely heated through.

Optional Extras

17. Greek yogurt to serve once cooked. Enjoy! ♥

Chicken and Roast Pepper Curry

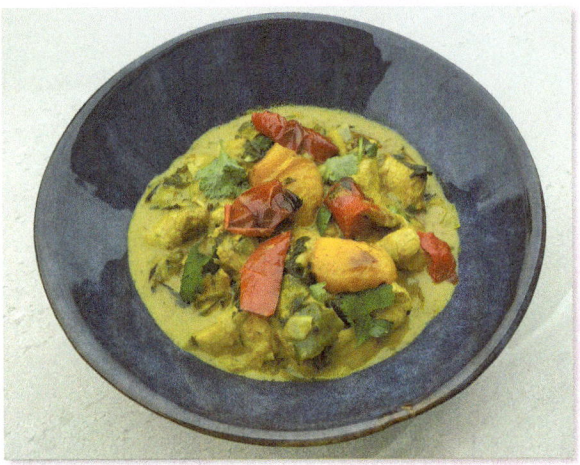

This is a super-easy follow-on from the curry base to create a lovely meal. As with all the curries, you can add any meat of your choice. If you don't eat meat, you could swap it for halloumi, paneer or boiled eggs.

Equipment
- Large saucepan
- Roasting dish or another large saucepan

Top Tips
- This **can** be frozen.

Making Time Approximately 45–50 minutes

Makes 4 portions

Per Portion
8.6g carbs / 39.1g protein / 476 calories / 31.9g fat

INGREDIENTS

The Base Recipe
- 1 batch curry (page 24)

The Rest of the Ingredients
- 600g chicken breast, chunky chopped
- 20g olive oil or coconut oil
- 300g peppers, chunky chopped

Optional Extra
- An extra 200ml coconut milk if you'd like it a little saucier

METHOD

The Base Recipe
1. Make the curry (page 24)

The Rest of the Recipe
2. Heat the oven to 190°C or the Ninja to 180°C.
3. Add the chicken to the base recipe, bring to a boil and then turn down to a simmer for about 20–30 minutes, or until the chicken is fully cooked. Pop the lid on to speed it up.
4. While the curry is cooking, move on to the peppers. You have two choices here: you can either fry or roast! If you're roasting, pop the oil and peppers into a casserole dish, mix well and roast in the oven for about 25 minutes or if you are cooking in the Ninja, for approx. 20 minutes. If you are frying, add the oil and peppers to a large pan and fry for approximately 10 minutes.
5. When the peppers are cooked, add them to the curry base and give it a good stir.
6. If you'd like a little more sauce add a splash of water or more coconut milk.
7. And that's it! Enjoy! ❤

One Curry Four Ways

Roast Vegetable and Butter Bean Curry

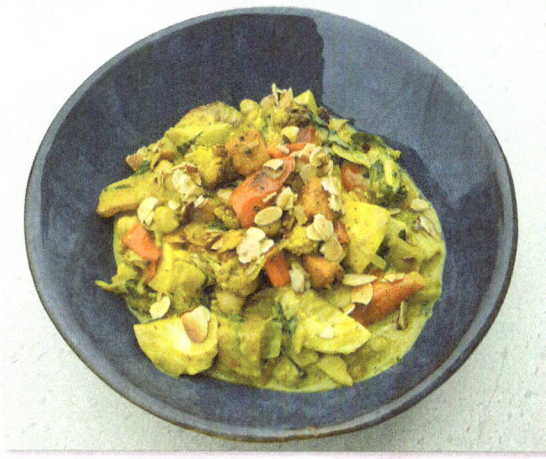

This is a lovely follow-on from the curry base to create a really tasty vegetarian meal. As with all the curries, you can add meat to this if you prefer and take the beans out to lower the carbs.

Equipment
- Large saucepan
- Large ovenproof dish

Top Tips
- This **can** be frozen, but **not** if you add boiled eggs. These can be added fresh after it's defrosted.

Making Time Approximately 45 minutes

Makes 4 portions

Per Portion
17.1g carbs / 9.1g protein / 542 calories / 48.8g fat

So the carbs are a little higher due to this being a vegetarian dish and the fact that it has 100g of butter beans. You can swap the butter beans for chickpeas or any bean of your choice, or just eliminate completely.

INGREDIENTS

The Base Recipe
- 1 batch curry (page 24)

The Rest of the Ingredients
- 200g cauliflower or broccoli, chunky chopped
- 100g peppers, chunky chopped
- 100g butternut squash or swede, chunky chopped (I've based the carbs on swede)
- 30g coconut oil
- 50g flaked almonds
- 2 teaspoons curry powder
- Salt and pepper (I add ½ teaspoon salt and ¼ teaspoon freshly ground black pepper)
- 200ml coconut milk
- 100g butter beans

Optional Extra
For extra protein add 8 boiled eggs (2 per portion). The extra macros per portion will be 132 calories / 0.0g carbs / 13g protein / 8.8g fat

METHOD

The Base Recipe
1. Make the curry (page 24)

The Rest of the Recipe
2. Heat the oven to 190°C or the Ninja to 180°C.
3. In an ovenproof dish, add cauliflower, peppers, swede, oil, flaked almonds, curry powder and seasoning. Give it a good mix and pop in the oven for about 20–25 minutes.
4. Optional eggs. *While the vegetables and base are cooking, boil your eggs. I start my eggs in cold water. When the water is boiling, set the timer for 6 minutes. Empty the water and add cold water, then peel the shells. Chunky chop the eggs.*
5. When the vegetables in the oven are cooked, add them to the curry base, along with the coconut milk, boiled eggs and butter beans and heat through.
6. And that's it! Enjoy! ♥

Chicken, Tomato and Roast Vegetables Curry

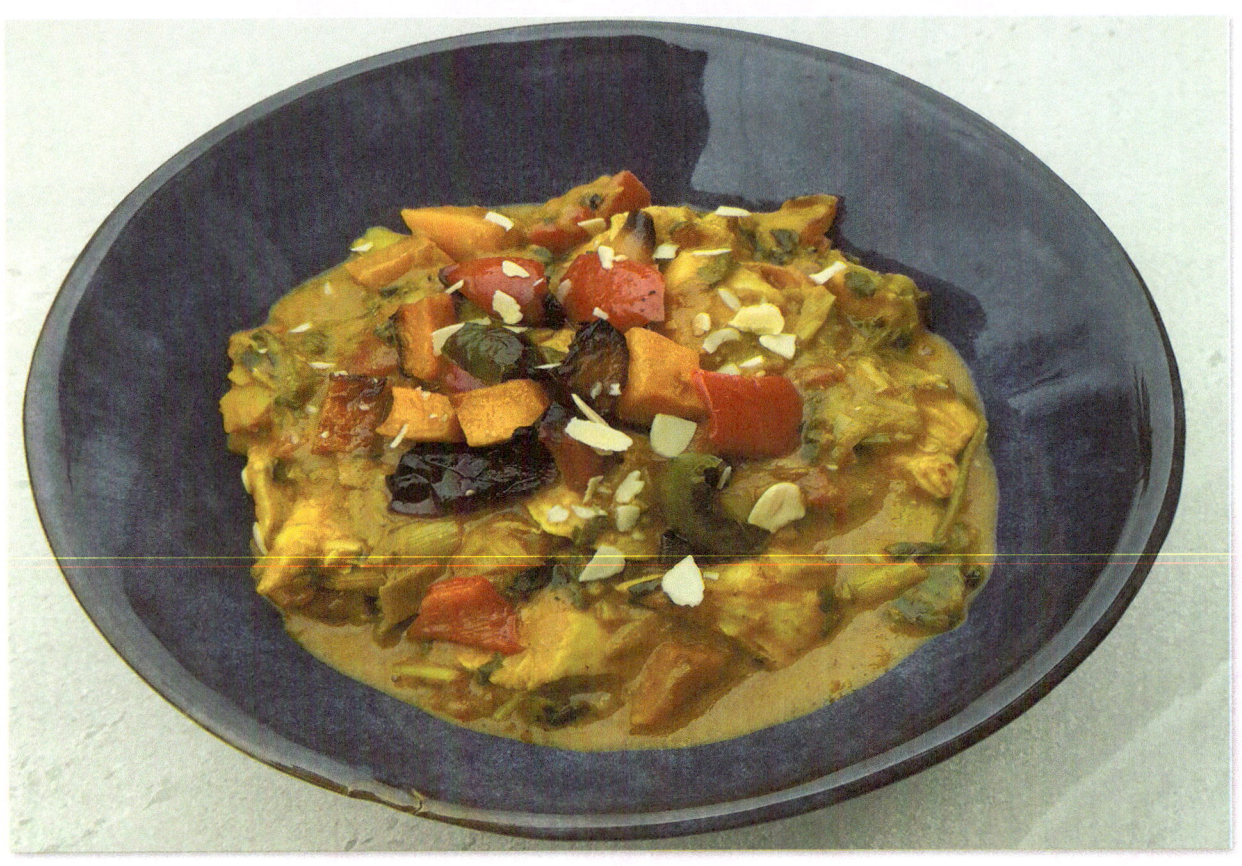

This is another easy follow-on from the curry base to create a lovely nutritional meal. As with all the curries, you can add any meat of your choice. If you don't eat meat, swap it for a bit of halloumi, paneer or boiled eggs.

Equipment
- Large non-stick saucepan
- Ovenproof dish

Top Tips
- This **can** be frozen.

Making Time
Approximately 45 minutes

Makes
4 portions

Per Portion
14g carbs / 40.1g protein / 500 calories / 31.9g fat

INGREDIENTS

The Base Recipe
- 1 batch curry (page 24)

The Rest of the Ingredients
- 600g chicken breast, chunky chopped
- 400g tinned tomatoes (good quality)
- 200g swede or butternut squash, chunky chopped
- 100g peppers, chunky chopped
- 20g olive oil or coconut oil

METHOD

The Base Recipe
1. Make the curry (page 24)

The Rest of the Recipe
2. Heat the oven to 190°C or the Ninja to 180°C.
3. Add the chicken and tinned tomatoes to the base recipe (put a little water in the empty tin and give a little clean and add this to the curry too), bring to a boil and then turn down to a gentle simmer for about 20–30 minutes, or until the chicken is fully cooked. Pop the lid on to speed it up.
4. Meanwhile, in an ovenproof dish, add the swede, peppers and oil. Give them a good mix and pop in the oven for about 20–25 minutes.
5. Once the vegetables are cooked, add them to the base recipe, which already has the tinned tomatoes and chicken added. Give it a good stir.
6. And that's it! Enjoy! ♥

One Pie Crust
Four Ways

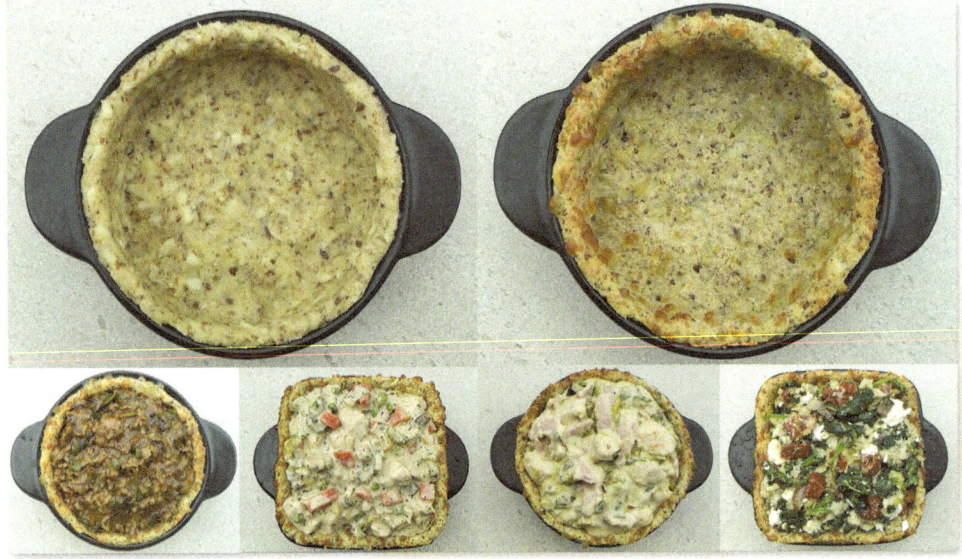

What is this crust? I would say it's a cross between a pastry and bread. Soft in the middle and crusty on the outside.

This is a high-fat, high-calorie recipe. So to help you decide, in each recipe it has 3 macro sections, four-portions, six-portions and fillings-only macros.

Equipment
- Large bowl
- Rolling pin
- Silicone sheets or silicone rolling mat (page xvi)
- 1 large pie dish or 4/6 smaller pie dishes. This pastry is very forgiving, so find the size of dish that works for you.

Top Tips
- Wet your hands while working this dough; it's very sticky.
- Olive oil your rolling pin and rolling/silicon mat too.
- This **can** be frozen.

Making Time Approximately 20 minutes

Makes 4 / 6 portions

Per Portion
6.8g carbs / 25.5g protein / 639 calories / 53.9g fat (*if 4 portions*)
4.5g carbs / 17g protein / 426 calories / 36g fat (*if 6 portions*)

Four Ways
Beef and leek pie (page 34); Chicken and vegetable in gravy pie (page 36); Creamy chicken and ham Pie (page 38); Spinach and feta pie (page 40)

INGREDIENTS
- 130g ground almonds
- 130g milled golden linseed
- 20g psyllium husk
- 2 teaspoons xanthan gum
- ½ teaspoon salt
- 50g melted butter, cooled
- 100g cream cheese
- 4 eggs

TOPPING
- 50g mature cheddar, grated

METHOD
1. Heat the oven to 190°C or the Ninja to 180°C.
2. Add all the dry ingredients, excluding the cheddar to a large bowl and mix.
3. Add all the wet ingredients to the dry mix, and stir well until you have a nice wet dough. Allow to rest for a couple of minutes.
4. Divide the dough into two-thirds (base) and one-third (topping).
5. Grease your dish or dishes well, and roll out the two-thirds dough between two pieces of greaseproof paper or silicone paper until it fits your dish or dishes.
6. Line your dish with the rolled-out dough. Neaten the edges and patchwork any gaps if needed. If you have problems transferring the dough, keep it on the greaseproof paper and flip it upside down into the base of your dish while still attached to the paper. Gently peel away the paper.
7. Bake in the oven for about 10 minutes or in the Ninja for about 5 minutes. Do not brown it; just crisp it up a little.
8. Pop in your chosen pie filling:
   - Beef and leek pie (page 34)
   - Chicken and vegetable in gravy pie (page 36)
   - Creamy chicken and ham pie (page 38)
   - Spinach and feta pie (page 40).
9. Roll out the remaining one-third dough and pop this over your pie filling. Seal the edges and sprinkle over the grated cheese.
   If you'd like to freeze it, then it can be frozen at this stage. Defrost and cook for approximately 30 minutes.
10. Bake for a further (approximately) 20 minutes. Basically, until the top crust is crispy and the filling is between 73°C and 83°C.
11. This can be frozen before or after baking the top. Enjoy! ♥

Beef and Leek in Gravy Pie

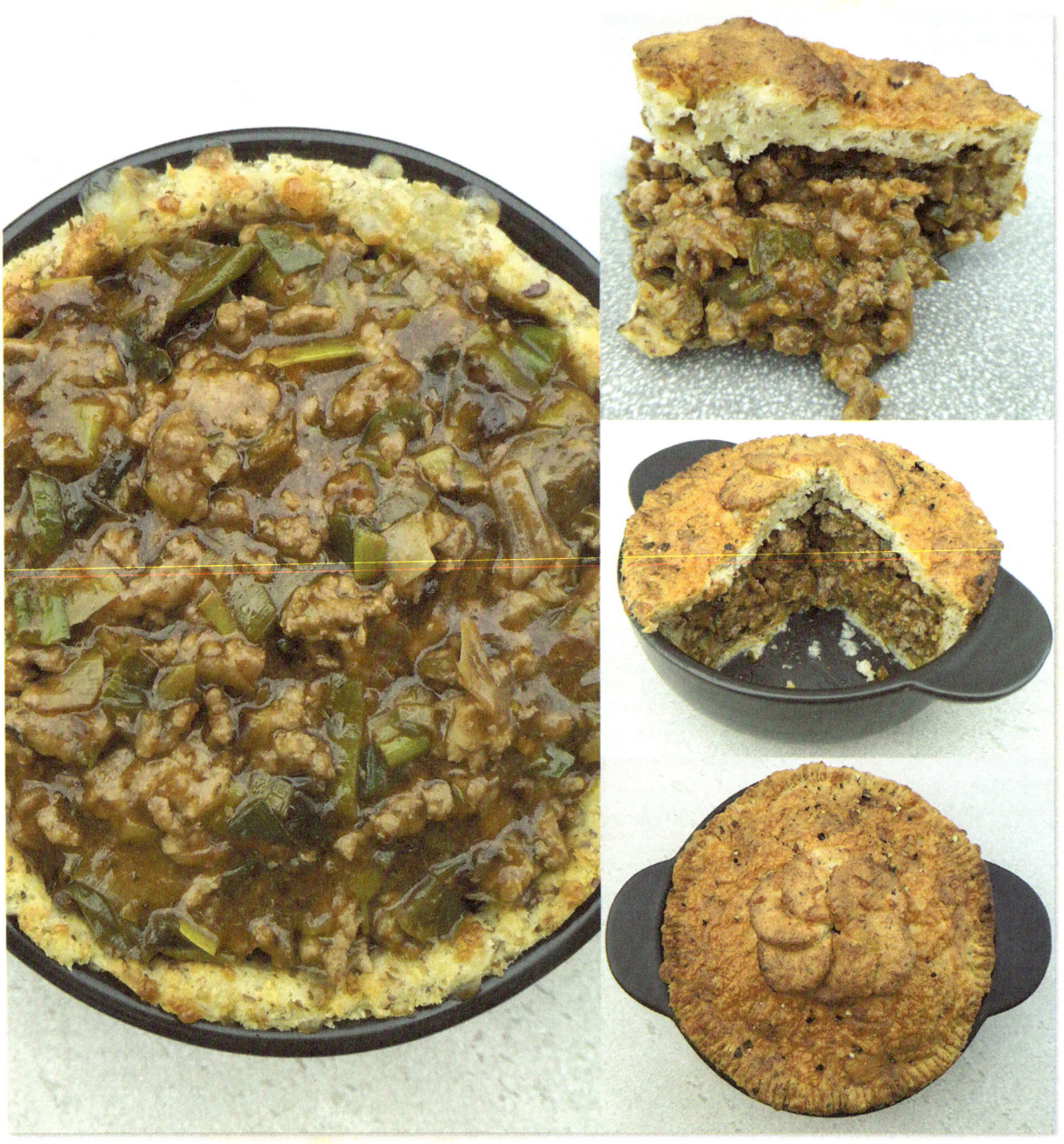

I don't like to admit to having a favourite… but, yes, this is the one!

Equipment
- Large bowl
- Rolling pin
- Silicone sheets or silicone rolling mat (page xvi)
- Saucepan

Top Tips
- This **can** be frozen.

Making Time
Approximately 45 minutes

Makes
4 / 6 portions

Per Portion
17.1g carbs / 58.9g protein / 919 calories / 66g fat (*if 4 portions*)
11.4g carbs / 39.2g protein / 613 calories / 44g fat (*if 6 portions*)
41.1g carbs / 133.3g protein / 1123 calories / 48.3g fat (*pie filling only*)

INGREDIENTS

The Base Recipe
- 1 batch pie crust (page 32)

The Filling
- 20g olive oil
- 300g leeks, small roughly chopped
- 600g beef mince
- 2 teaspoons garlic purée or 3 garlic cloves, finely chopped
- 10–15g arrowroot
- 2 tablespoons Worcestershire sauce
- 20g tomato puree
- 2 teaspoons mixed herbs
- 2 beef stock cubes
- 150–200ml boiling water (or whatever is needed to give you the right amount of gravy—my husband wanted more, which is why I have upped it to 200ml)
- Salt and pepper (I added ½ teaspoon salt and ¼ teaspoon freshly ground black pepper)

METHOD

The Base Recipe
1. Make the pie crust (page 32)

The Pie Filling
1. Add the oil to a large pan and fry the leeks for about 5–10 minutes until they are softened but not browned—almost translucent.
2. Now add the beef mince and garlic and fry until the beef is lightly cooked but not crispy.
3. Next add the arrowroot, Worcestershire Sauce, tomato puree and mixed herbs and stir through.
4. Finally, add the stock cubes and boiling water to the saucepan and season with salt and pepper.
5. Bring to a boil and then turn down to a gentle simmer for approximately 15–20 minutes.
6. Simmer for longer if you want to reduce the gravy; or if you like the gravy as it is but would like it a little thicker, add a small amount of extra arrowroot to a cup, with a little cold water, mix until smooth and then mix into the pie filling.
7. Now pour into your prepared pie crust base and go back to the pie crust recipe (page 32) and continue to follow the instructions from **Step 9** onwards. Enjoy! ♥

Chicken and Vegetable in Gravy Pie

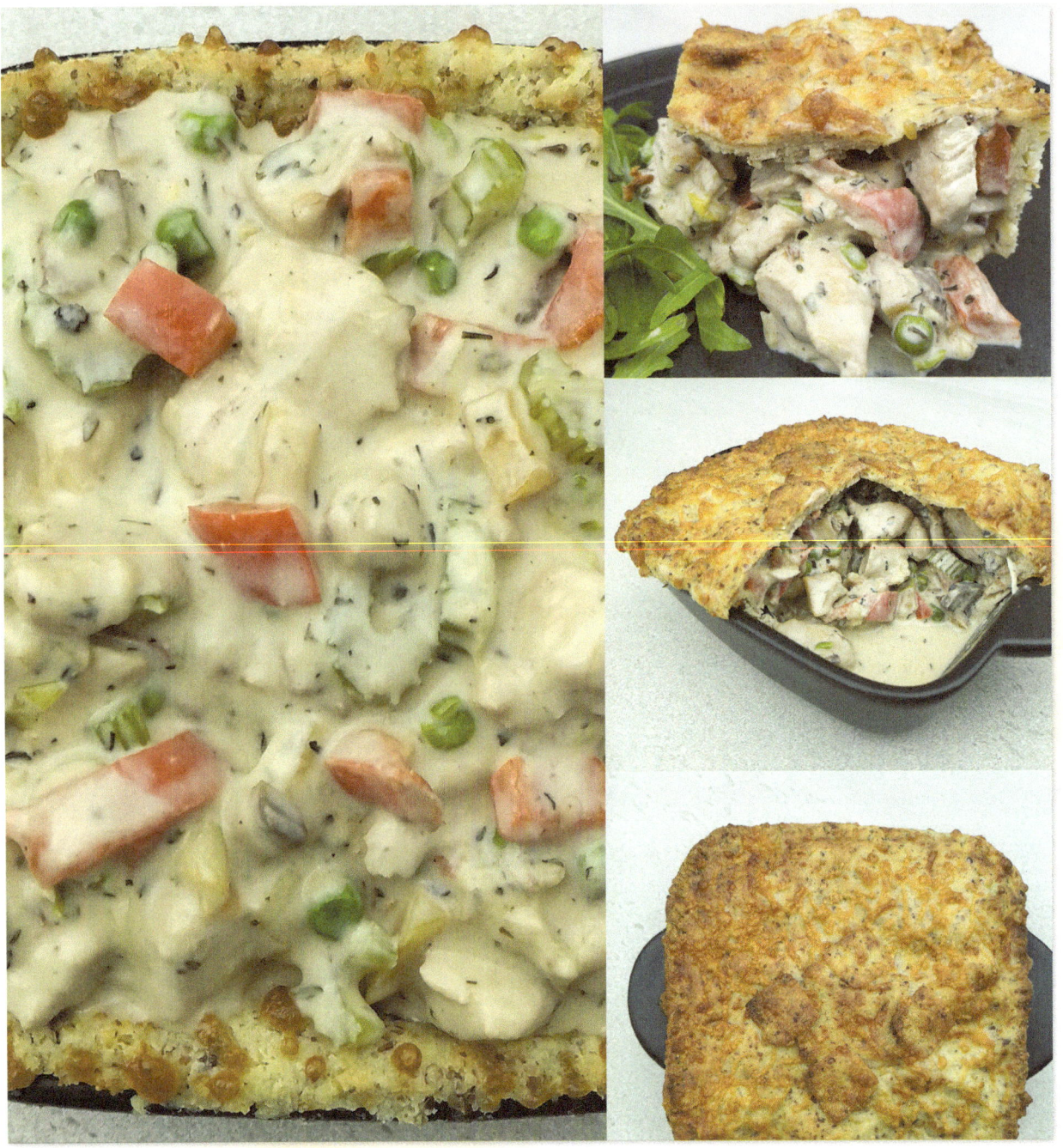

I particularly love this pie because it has everything my boys love about a pie: chicken, vegetables and gravy. Oh, and it's super filling.

Equipment
- Large bowl
- Rolling pin
- Silicone sheets or silicone rolling mat (page xvi)
- Saucepan

Top tips
- This **can** be frozen.

Making Time
Approximately 45 minutes

Makes
4 / 6 portions

Per Portion
14.5g carbs / 64.4g protein / 1030 calories / 77.3g fat (*if 4 portions*)
9.5g carbs / 42.9g protein / 686 calories / 51.5g fat (*if 6 portions*)
29.7g carbs / 155.4g protein / 1564 calories / 93.4g fat (*pie filling only*)

INGREDIENTS

The Base Recipe
- 1 batch pie crust (page 32)

The Filling
The chicken and all the vegetables to be small roughly chopped, apart from the peas!

- 100g swede
- 40g butter
- 100g leeks
- 600g chicken
- 100g peppers
- 100g celery
- 100g mushrooms
- ½ teaspoon garlic paste or 1 garlic clove, finely chopped
- 2 teaspoons dried mixed herbs
- 2 chicken stock cubes
- 300ml boiling water
- Salt and pepper (I add ½ teaspoon salt and ¼ teaspoon freshly ground black pepper)
- 100ml double cream
- 50g frozen peas

Optional extra thickener
- 15g arrowroot, made up with 30ml of cold water or milk

METHOD

The Base Recipe
1. Make the pie crust (page 32)

The Filling
1. Pop the swede in a microwave bowl with a little water and microwave for about 5–7 minutes. This is to speed up the cooking time of this vegetable, as the swede takes the longest to cook.
2. Add the butter to a large pan and fry the leeks for about 5 minutes until they are softened but not browned (almost translucent).
3. Now add the chicken and fry for a further 5 minutes.
4. Add the swede and all the other vegetables, apart from the peas.
5. Add the garlic and herbs and stir through and fry for a further 5 minutes.
6. Add the stock cubes, boiling water and seasoning to the pan.
7. Allow to simmer for about 20–30 minutes until all the vegetables are cooked.
8. Add the cream and peas and stir through.
9. Simmer for longer if you want to reduce the gravy; or if you like the gravy as it is but would like it a little thicker, add a small amount of arrowroot to a cup, with a little cold water, mix until smooth and then mix into the pie filling.
10. Now pour into your prepared pie crust base and go back to the pie crust recipe on page 32 and follow the instructions from **Step 9** onwards. Enjoy!

Creamy Chicken and Ham Pie

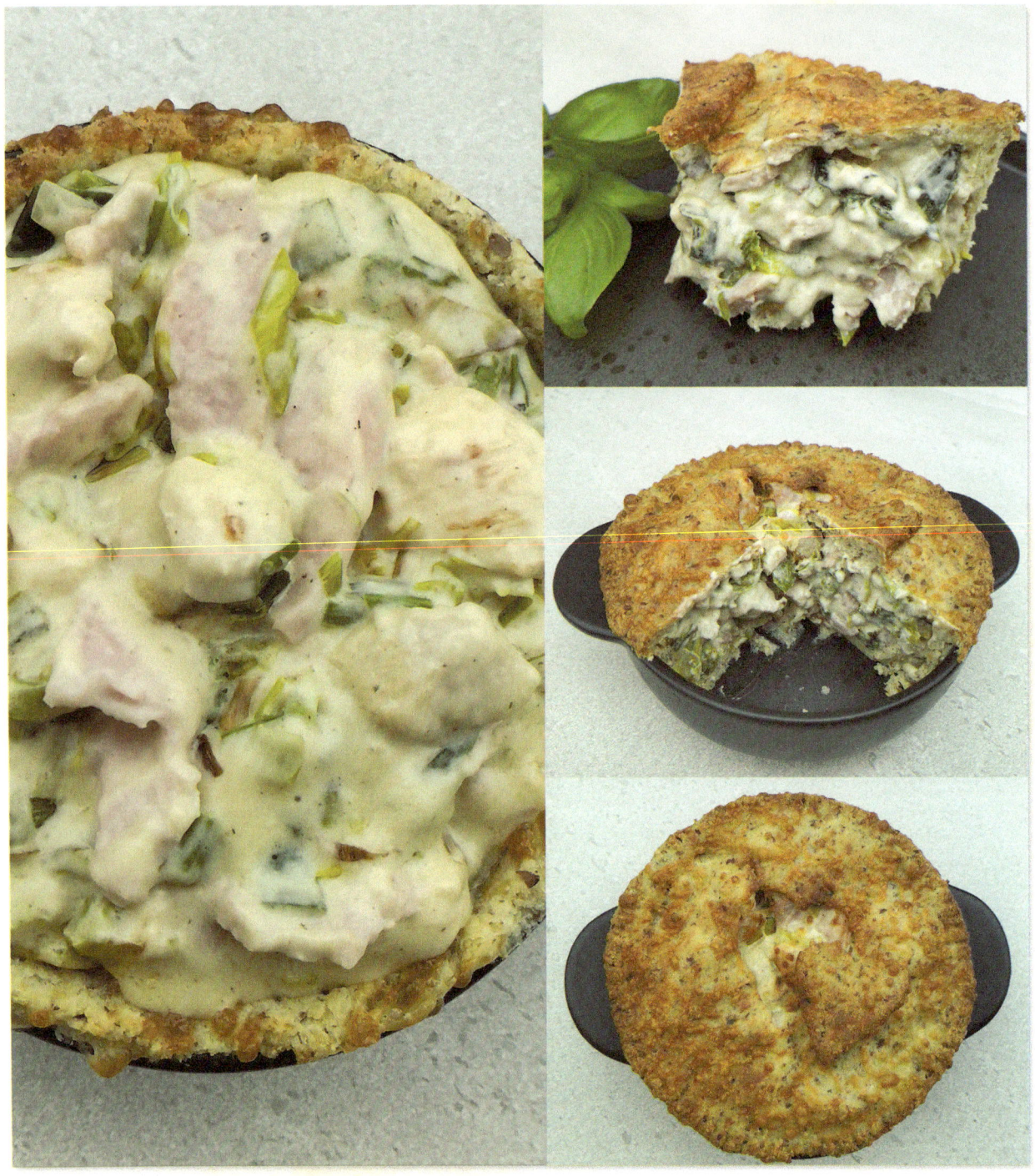

This is my son Ollie's second favourite of the four pies. His favourite is the chicken and vegetable in gravy.

38 One Pie Crust **Four Ways**

Equipment
- Large bowl
- Rolling pin
- Silicone sheets or silicone rolling mat (page xvi)
- Saucepan

Top Tips
- This **can** be frozen.

Making Time
Approximately 45 minutes

Makes
4/ 6 portions

Per Portion
18g carbs / 66.4g protein /1153 calories /88.1g fat (*if 4 portions*)
12g carbs / 44.3g protein / 769 calories / 58.7g fat (*if 6 portions*)
44.7g carbs / 163.6g protein / 2057 calories / 136.6g fat (*pie filling only*)

INGREDIENTS

The Base Recipe
- 1 batch pie crust (page 32)

The Filling
- 20g butter
- 20g olive oil
- 300g leeks, small roughly chopped
- 400g chicken, small roughly chopped chunks
- 200g cooked ham or gammon, small roughly chopped chunks
- ½ teaspoon garlic paste or 1 garlic clove, crushed or finely chopped
- 250ml milk (I like to use full-fat lactose-free milk, which the macros are based on)
- 150ml double cream
- 1 chicken stock cube
- 20g parmesan, finely grated
- Salt and pepper (I add ½ teaspoon salt and ¼ teaspoon freshly ground black pepper)
- 20g arrowroot (mixed with 30ml cold water to create a thickening agent)

The Optional Extra
- Ready-grated mozzarella (to thicken the sauce in place of the arrowroot; it will increase the fat, but lower the carbs)

METHOD

The Base Recipe
1. Make the pie crust (page 32)

The Filling
2. Add the butter and olive oil to a large pan and fry the leeks for about 5–10 minutes until they are softened but not browned (almost translucent).
3. Now add the chicken and fry until cooked (about 5–10 minutes).
4. Add all the remaining ingredients, **apart from the arrowroot mixed with water**, stir well and bring up to almost bubbling, then turn down to a gentle simmer.
5. Now add the arrowroot and stir through the sauce in the pan. Allow to thicken. If you'd like it a little thicker, either add more arrowroot, mixed with a little water in the same way, or, if you'd like to keep the carbs lower, add a sprinkling of ready-grated mozzarella and stir through until it thickens.
6. Now pour into your prepared pie crust base and go back to the pie crust recipe on page 32 and follow the instructions from **Step 9** onwards. Enjoy! ♥

Spinach and Feta Pie

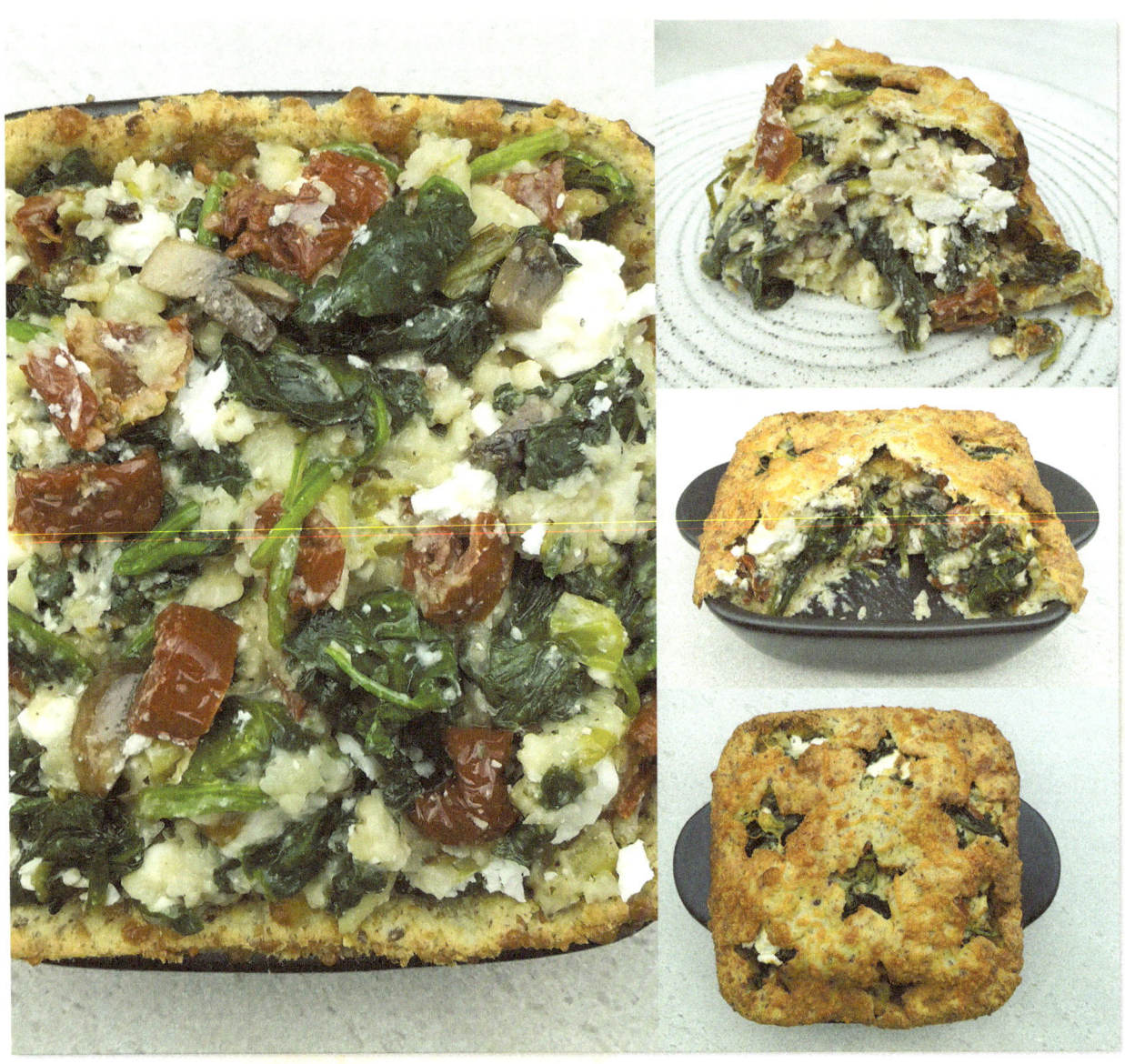

One of my Cypriot friends inspired me to make this dish ... although it's actually based on a Greek dish that has a filo-pastry topping. I loved the idea of a pie filled with mash, but in this pie I have used celeriac mash instead. If you're not too fond of celeriac, why not try swede? Just make sure you overcook the swede, to make the perfect mash.

Equipment
- Large bowl
- Rolling pin
- Silicone sheets or silicone rolling mat (page xvi)
- Saucepan

Top Tips
- This **can** be frozen.

Making Time
Approximately 45 minutes

Makes
4 / 6 portions

Per Portion
14.5g carbs / 45.1g protein / 1066 calories / 88.8g fat (*if 4 portions*)
9.7g carbs / 30.1g protein / 710 calories / 59.2g fat (*if 6 portions*)
30.8g carbs / 78.5g protein / 1708 calories / 139.6g fat (*pie filling only*)

INGREDIENTS

The Base Recipe
- 1 batch pie crust (page 32)

The Mash Filling
- 400g celeriac, small roughly chopped
- 20g butter
- Salt and pepper (I add ½ teaspoon salt and ¼ teaspoon freshly ground black pepper)

The Rest of the Filling
All the vegetables, including the sundried tomatoes, small roughly chopped.

- 30g olive oil
- 100g leeks
- 100g mushrooms
- 2 teaspoons garlic paste or 3 garlic cloves, crushed or finely chopped
- 400g spinach
- 200g feta
- 100g sundried tomatoes
- 100g cheddar, grated
- 2 teaspoons dried oregano/mixed herbs
- Salt and pepper (I add ½ teaspoon salt and ¼ teaspoon freshly ground black pepper)

METHOD

The Base Recipe
1. Make the pie crust (page 32)

The Mash Filling
2. Start by boiling or steaming the celeriac or swede (I prefer to steam, as I really feel it keeps its full flavour). This will take about 15–20 minutes.
3. Once cooked, add all the mash ingredients to a food processor (this can be done with a potato masher too) and blitz until super smooth.
4. Put this to one side.

The Rest of the Filling
5. Meanwhile, in a large non-stick saucepan, add the olive oil and leeks and fry for about 5 minutes until translucent but not browned.
6. Add the mushrooms and fry for 2 minutes.
7. Now add the garlic and spinach and cook until the spinach has wilted. This will take all of 2–3 minutes.
8. Take off the heat and add all the other filling ingredients, including the mash, and mix well.
9. Now pour into your prepared pie crust base and go back to the pie crust recipe on page 32 and follow the instructions from **Step 9** onwards. Enjoy! ♥

One Rainbow Rice
Four Ways

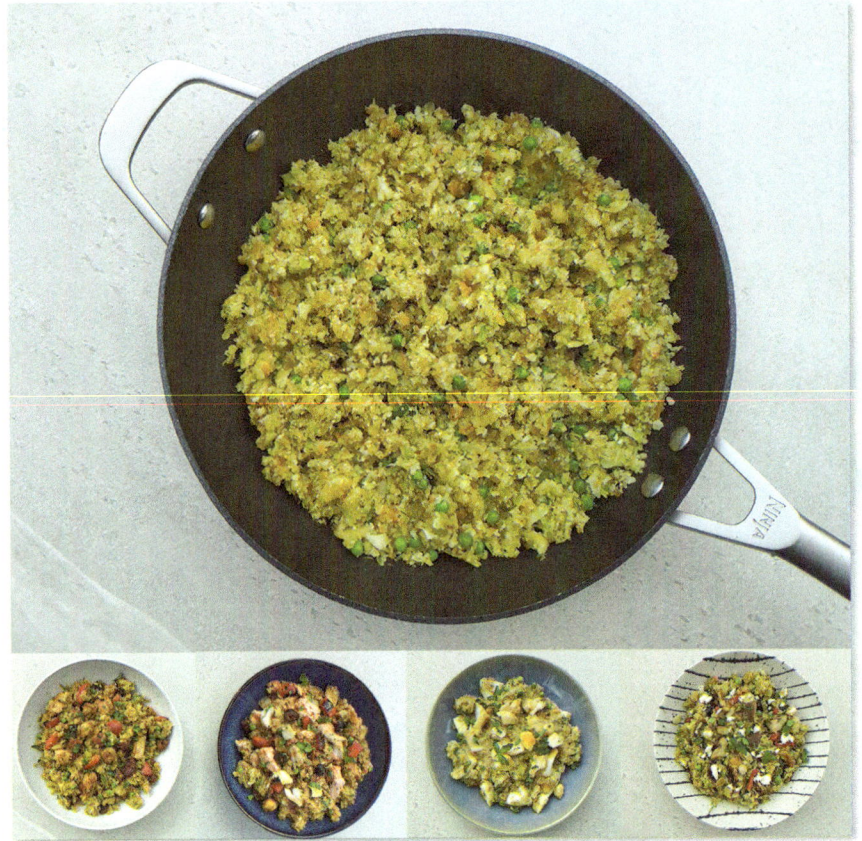

This is a really delicious recipe on its own. What can you do with this dish? Well, there are four fabulous recipes that really make a meal of this base recipe. But you could also just add some good-quality curry powder or a little turmeric and this will also make it into a beautiful side dish. Just add some protein and there's a fabulous nutritionally well-balanced meal. Or make a well in the centre of your rice pan and scramble some eggs and stir them through. A very quick egg-fried rice.

The beauty of this dish is that it's a really good way of using up out-of-date vegetables and the stalks. I've selected these vegetables, as these were what was in my fridge at the time of writing this recipe. But have a play; most low-carb vegetables will work. At the front of this book (page xiii) I have briefly explained about vegetable substitutions.

Equipment
- Food processor
- Large non-stick saucepan

Top Tips
- To reduce the carb content of this dish, you could switch the swede for more cauliflower or use broccoli stalks instead.
- This **can** be frozen.

Making Time
Approximately 45 minutes

Makes
4 portions

Per Portion
13.5g carbs / 4.9g protein / 137 calories / 7.6g fat

Four Ways
Chicken and chorizo (page 44); Fish paella (page 46); Kedgeree (page 48); Nutty vegetarian (page 50)

INGREDIENTS
- 400g cauliflower, chunky chopped
- 400g swede or butternut squash, chunky chopped (please note that using butternut squash will increase the carbs — macros have been calculated using swede)
- 150g leeks, chunky chopped
- 2 teaspoons garlic puree or 3 garlic cloves, finely chopped
- Salt and pepper (I add 1 teaspoon salt and ½ teaspoon freshly ground black pepper)
- 15g olive oil
- 15g butter (or coconut oil for dairy free)
- 1 vegetable stock cube
- 100ml boiling water
- 50g frozen peas

METHOD
1. In a food processor, blitz up the vegetables, garlic and seasoning until it resembles rice.
2. In a frying pan, melt the oil and butter.
3. Once it starts to sizzle, add all the ingredients, **apart** from the stock cube, water and peas.
4. Keep stirring and frying until all the vegetables are softened and cooked, but not browned. This will take about 10–15 minutes.
5. Meanwhile, make up your stock with 100ml boiling water and add your peas to the stock.
6. When the rainbow rice is cooked, add to this your stock and peas.
7. Stir until all the ingredients are well combined.
8. Your rainbow rice base is now ready
9. Enjoy this as it is or move on to the four other fabulous rice dishes.
10. **To reheat, either stir-fry or microwave. If reheating in the oven, make sure you cover the dish with foil, so it doesn't dry out.** Enjoy! ♥

Chicken and Chorizo

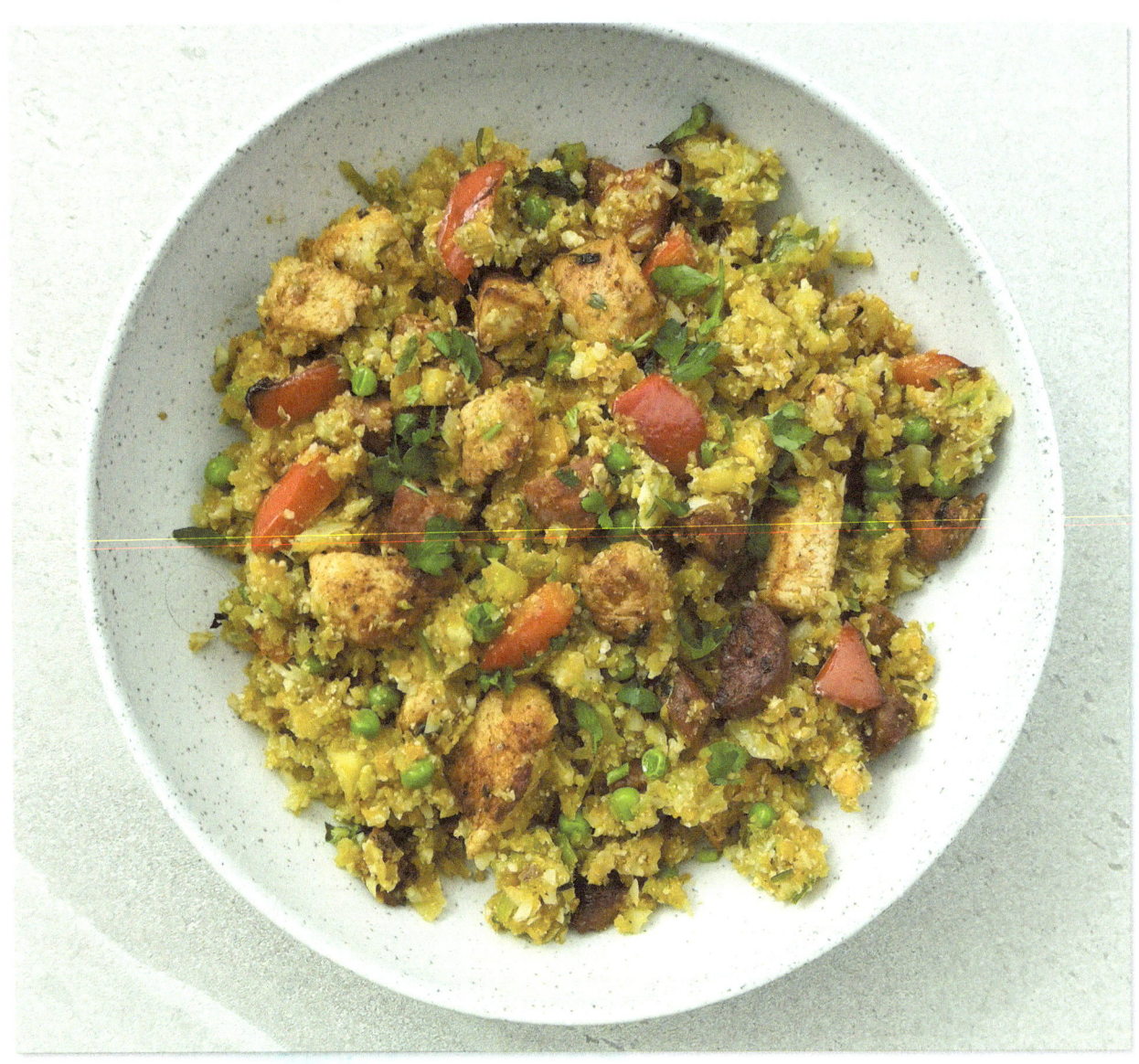

The natural oils that seep out of the chorizo when cooking adds wonderful extra flavour and a beautiful colour to the dish, so don't tip those juices away. Make sure you add it all to the rainbow rice.

Equipment
- Food processor
- Large non-stick saucepan

Top Tips
- This **can** be frozen.

Making Time
Approximately 45 minutes

Makes
4 portions

Per Portion
16.5g carbs / 41.5g protein / 494 calories / 29.7g fat

INGREDIENTS

The Base Recipe
- 1 batch rainbow rice (page 42)

The Rest of the Ingredients
- 400g chicken breast, chunky chopped
- 200g chorizo, chunky chopped
- 120g red pepper, chunky chopped
- 20g olive oil
- 2 teaspoons paprika
- 25g fresh, flat-leaf parsley, roughly chopped

METHOD

The Base Recipe
1. Make the rainbow rice (page 42)

The Rest of the Ingredients

2. Heat the oven to 180°C or the Ninja to 170°C, or this can be fried in a non-stick frying pan.
3. Add the chicken, chorizo, peppers, olive oil and paprika to a bowl.
4. Give it a good mix.
5. Put the chicken and chorizo mix into the oven for about 25–30 minutes or until the chicken is cooked.
6. Once cooked, add all the ingredients, including the fresh parsley, to the rainbow rice base recipe and stir through.
7. **To reheat, either stir-fry or microwave. If reheating in the oven, make sure you cover the dish with foil, so it doesn't dry out.** Enjoy! ♥

Fish Paella

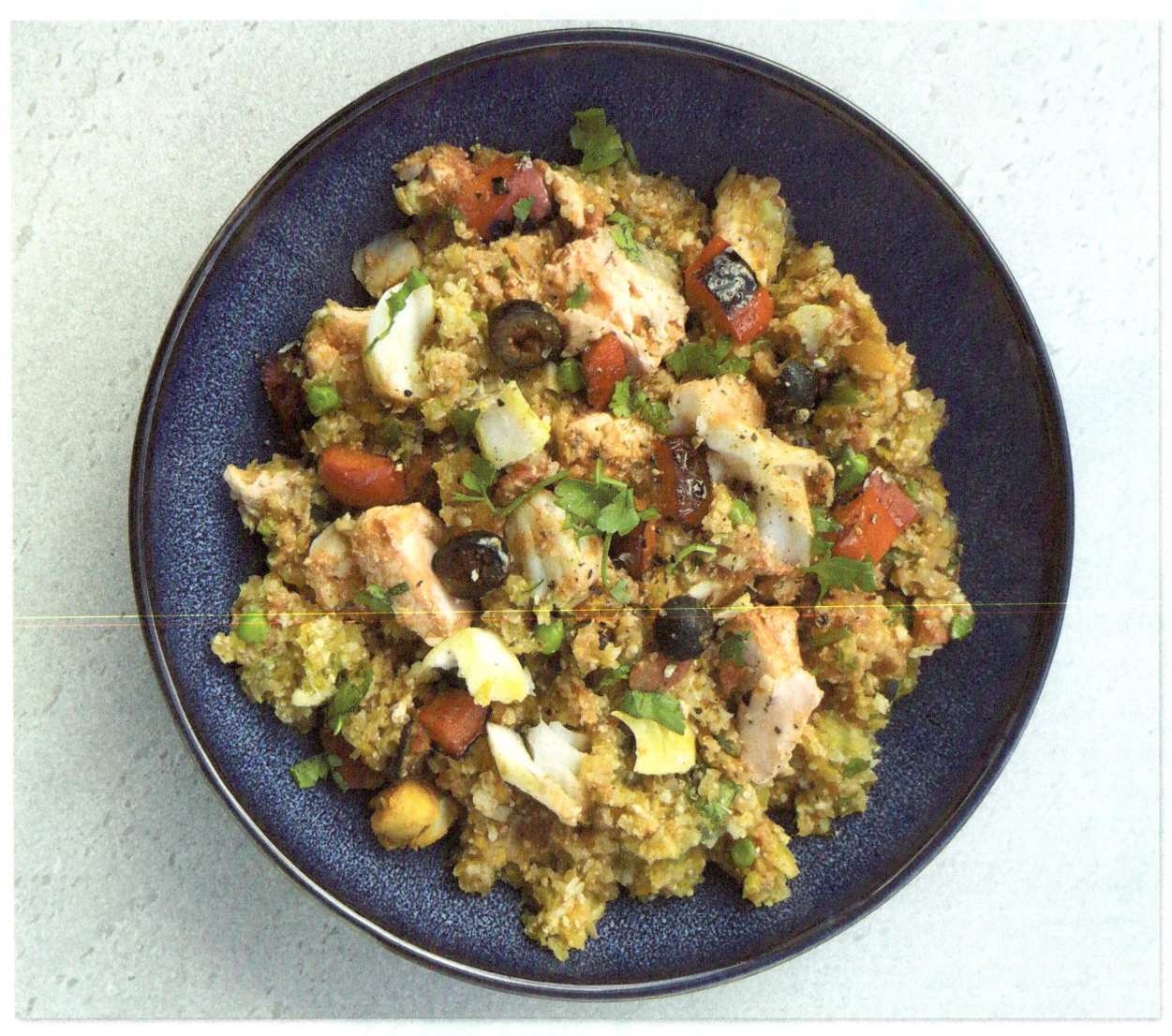

My favourite combination of fish is salmon, cod and haddock, and occasionally I'll throw in a handful of tiger prawns too. For a cheaper alternative, you can buy a bag of frozen mixed fish. In this case, I normally go for an 800g bag.

Equipment
- Food processor
- Large non-stick saucepan

Top Tips
- This **can** be frozen.

Making Time
Approximately 45 minutes

Makes
4 portions

Per Portion
20.3g carbs / 37.1g protein / 431 calories / 22.7g fat

INGREDIENTS
The Base Recipe
- 1 batch rainbow rice (page 42)

The Rest of the Ingredients
- 400g tinned tomatoes
- 50g olives, halved
- 3 teaspoons paprika
- 600g fish of your choice, or seafood mix (keep it whole, as it will naturally flake while cooking)
- 20g olive oil
- 200g red pepper, chunky chopped
- 25g fresh parsley
- 1 lemon (half to squeeze in the recipe and half to cut into 4 wedges)

METHOD
The Base Recipe
1. Make the rainbow ric)e (page 42).

The Rest of the Ingredients
2. In a non-stick saucepan, add the tinned tomatoes, olives, paprika and fish. Bring to a boil and then turn down to a gentle simmer until the fish is cooked through (approximately 15 minutes).
3. Meanwhile, in a frying pan, add the oil and heat up until sizzling, then add the peppers. Fry until completely cooked.
4. Once cooked, add all the ingredients, including the fresh parsley, to the rainbow rice base recipe and stir through.
5. **To reheat, either stir-fry or microwave. If reheating in the oven, make sure you cover the dish with foil, so it doesn't dry out.** Enjoy! ♥

Kedgeree

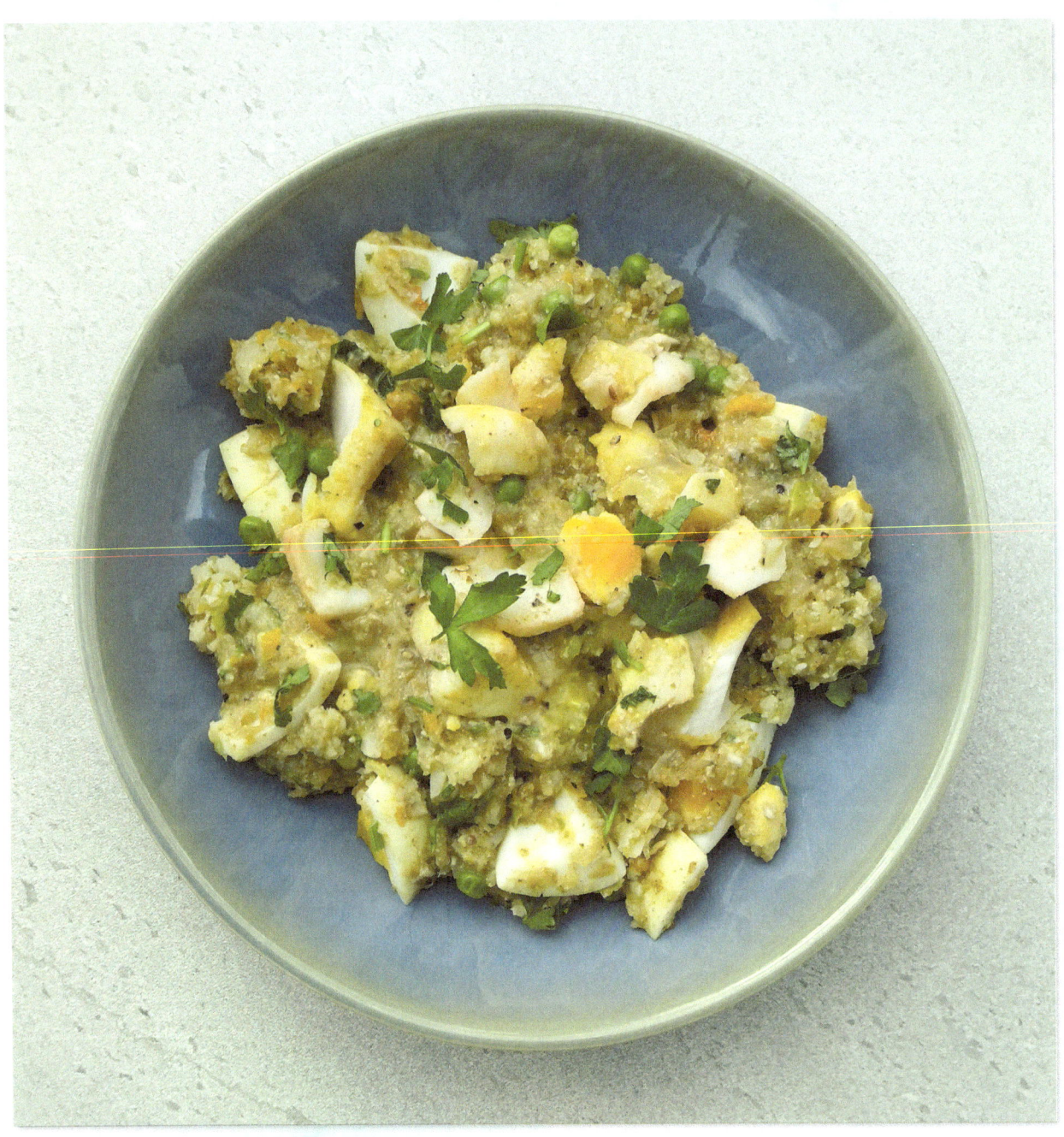

Call me an egg fan, but I love eggs! To freeze this recipe, leave out the eggs, and then add freshly boiled eggs after defrosting, following **Steps 4 and 5** when reheating.

Equipment
- Food processor
- Large non-stick saucepan

Top Tips
- This **cannot** be frozen, unless you add the boiled eggs fresh, after defrosting.

Making Time
Approximately 45 minutes

Makes
4 portions

Per Portion
18.5g carbs / 29.4g protein / 496 calories / 34.5g fat

INGREDIENTS

The Base Recipe
- 1 batch rainbow rice (page 42)

The Rest of the Ingredients
- 400 ml coconut milk
- 2 teaspoons curry powder
- 300g smoked haddock (leave the fish whole, as it will naturally break up while cooking and when you stir it through the rice)
- 20g olive oil
- 1 teaspoon curry powder – this is for the eggs
- 1½ teaspoons garlic puree or 2 garlic cloves, finely chopped
- 1½ teaspoons ginger puree or 2 teaspoons fresh ginger, finely chopped
- 4 boiled eggs
- 25g fresh parsley, chunky chopped

METHOD

The Base Recipe
1. Make the rainbow rice (page 42)

The Rest of the Ingredients
2. Add the coconut milk, curry powder (2 teaspoons) and haddock to a non-stick saucepan.
3. Bring the ingredients to almost boiling and then turn down to a gentle simmer. Simmer until all the fish is cooked, stirring occasionally. This will take about 10–15 minutes.
4. Meanwhile in another pan add the olive oil, curry powder (1 teaspoon), garlic and ginger and mix. Heat the pan up until the oil starts to bubble.
5. Add the whole boiled eggs and fry for 1 minute, then remove the pan from the heat and chunky chop the eggs.
6. Now add all of the remaining ingredients, including the fresh parsley, the juices from the egg pan and the contents of the fish pan to the rainbow rice base recipe and stir through.
7. **To reheat, either stir-fry or microwave. If reheating in the oven, make sure you cover the dish with foil, so it doesn't dry out.** Enjoy! ♥

Nutty Vegetarian

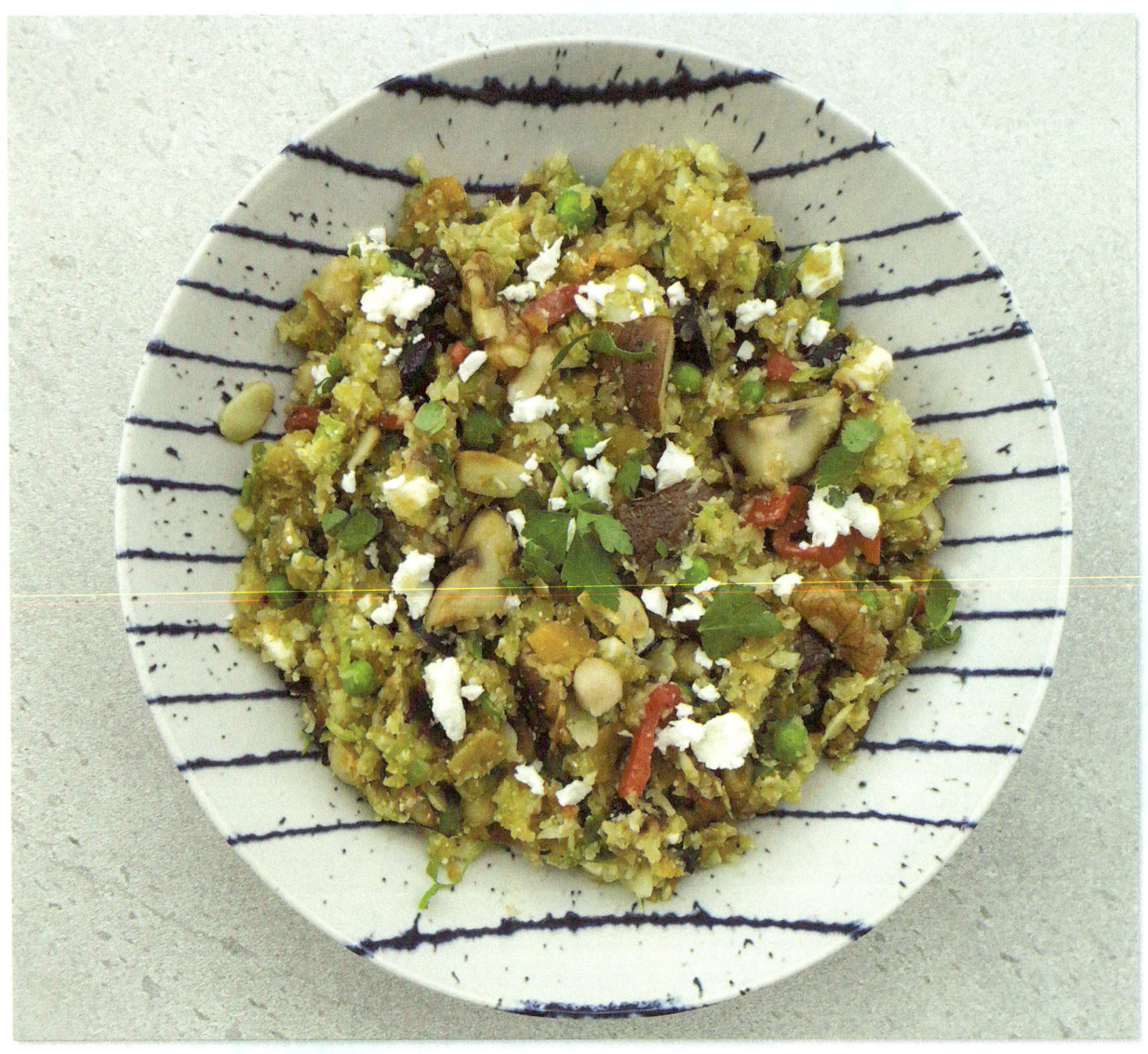

A delightful vegetarian version of the rainbow rice. This recipe is a higher-carb meal than all the other rice dishes.

Equipment
- Food processor
- Large non-stick saucepan

Top Tips
- This **can** be frozen.

Making Time
45 minutes

Makes
4 portions

Per Portion
21.3g carbs / 19.6g protein / 547 calories / 43.3g fat

INGREDIENTS

The Base Recipe
- 1 batch rainbow rice (page 42)

The Rest of the Ingredients
- 15g butter
- 15g olive oil
- 300g mushrooms, chunky chopped
- 50g walnuts, roughly chopped
- 50g flaked almonds
- 100g chickpeas
- 50g sundried tomatoes, chunky chopped
- 50g pitted olives, halved
- 100ml vegetable stock
- 25g fresh parsley, roughly chopped, or approximately 2 teaspoons dried parsley (half to mix in the recipe and half to sprinkle on top)
- 1 lemon (half to squeeze in the recipe and half to cut into 4 wedges)
- 100g blue cheese or feta

METHOD

The Base Recipe
1. Make the rainbow rice (page 42)

The Rest of the Ingredients
2. Add the olive oil and butter to a non-stick frying pan. Heat up until sizzling.
3. Add the mushrooms and fry for 5 minutes, then add the walnuts and flaked almonds and fry for a further 3 minutes.
4. Now add all the ingredients to the base recipe, apart from half of the parsley and the blue cheese. Give it a good stir.
5. Crumble in the cheese and gently stir in. Season more if needed.
6. Sprinkle the remaining parsley on top.
7. **To reheat, either stir-fry or microwave. If reheating in the oven, make sure you cover the dish with foil, so it doesn't dry out.**
Enjoy! ♥

One Salsa Four Ways

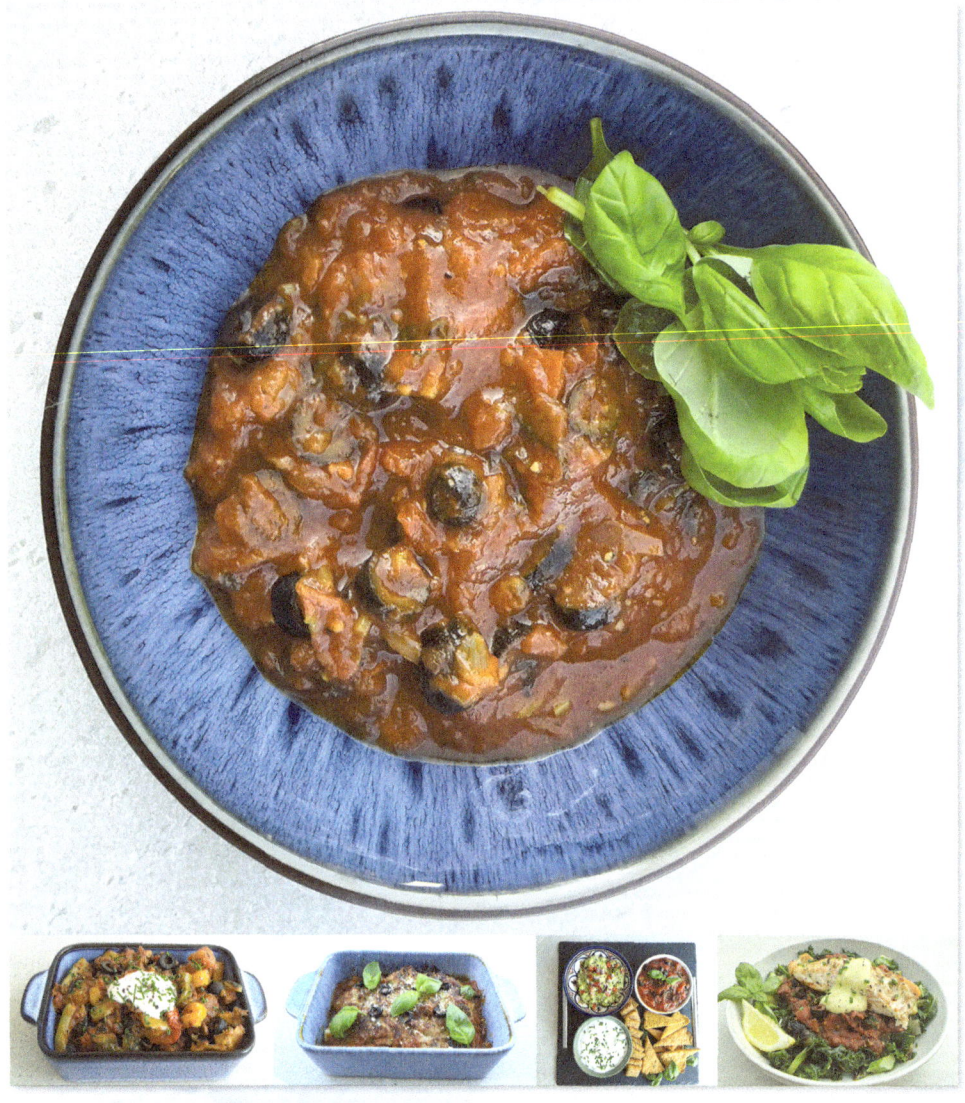

This dish has so many possibilities. As salsa, you can serve it hot or cold. My dear vegetarian friend would suggest swapping all meat for halloumi, 'As life is so much better with halloumi. So add halloumi!'

Equipment
- A small non-stick saucepan

Top Tips
- Sun dried tomatoes are a lovely alternative to olives.
- This **can** be frozen.

Making Time
Approx. 15 minutes

Four Ways
Baked vegetables and chorizo (page 54); Chicken and parmesan (page 56); Salmon and green vegetable parcel (page 58); Tortilla chips and three Mexican dips (page 60)

Makes
4 / 6 portions

Per Portion
4.7 g carbs / 1.9 g protein / 91 calories / 6.8 g fat (*if 4 portions*)
3.1 g carbs / 1.3 g protein / 60 calories / 4.5 g fat (*if 6 portions*)

INGREDIENTS
- 20g olive oil
- 25g shallots or 30g red onion, finely chopped
- 1½ teaspoons garlic puree or 2–3 garlic cloves, finely chopped
- 50g black or green pitted olives (or sun dried tomatoes), thinly sliced
- ½ teaspoon Kashmiri chilli powder or a medium chilli powder (start with ¼ teaspoon and see how spicy you prefer it, or you could swap the olive oil for Will's Chilli Oil (page 106)
- 1 teaspoon paprika
- 400g tinned tomatoes (good quality)
- 10g fresh basil or approximately ¾ teaspoon dried basil (**save half for the final step**)
- Salt and pepper (season well — I use ½ teaspoon salt and ¼ teaspoon freshly ground black pepper)
- ½ teaspoon sweetener (I like to use Truvia brown sweetener)

METHOD
1. In a non-stick saucepan, heat up the oil until sizzling.
2. Add the shallots or onions and lightly fry for about 5 minutes or until translucent, but not brown.
3. Then add the garlic, olives, Kashmiri chilli and paprika and gently fry for a further minute.
4. Add the tinned tomatoes.
5. Add **half** of the basil leaves, roughly torn up, plus the stems, finely chopped.
6. Add the seasoning and sweetener.
7. Bring to a boil and then turn down to a gentle simmer for about 10–15 minutes or until the salsa has reduced and thickened.
7. Finally, add the remaining basil leaves and stir in. Enjoy! ♥

Baked Vegetables and Chorizo

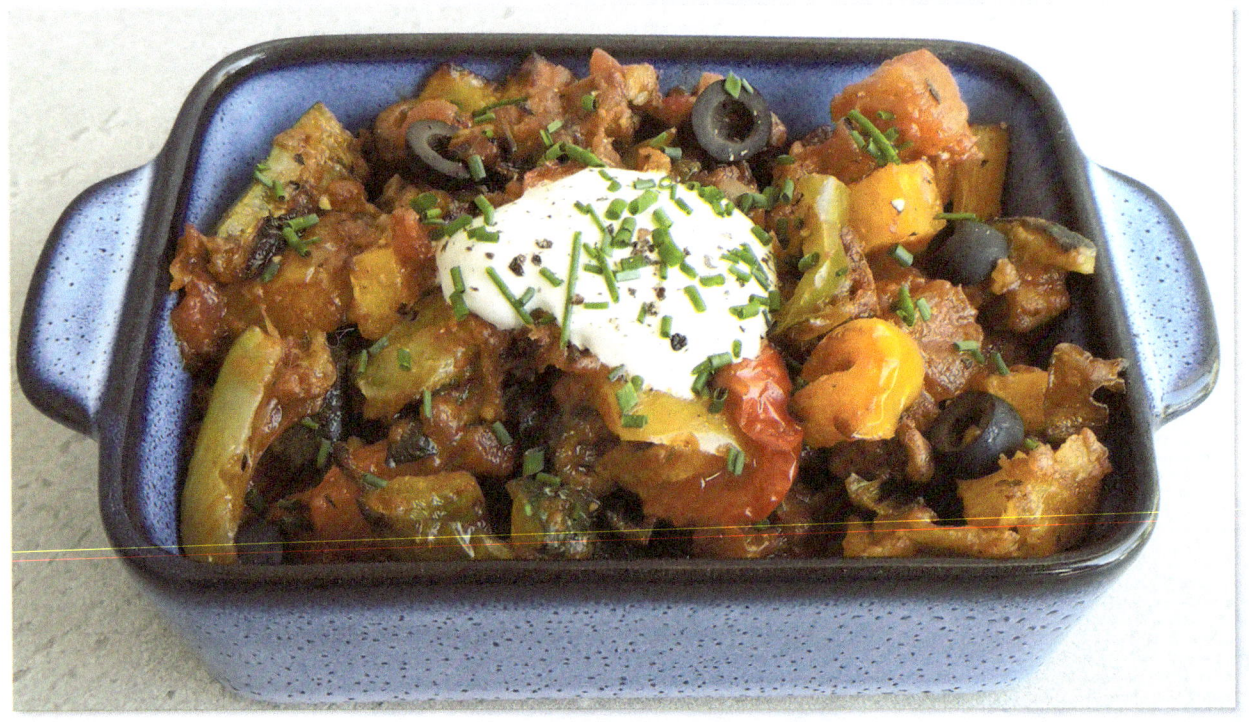

This dish will work with all sorts of vegetables; just work with whatever low-carb vegetables you have in your fridge.

Equipment
- Either a large saucepan or a large oven tray

Top Tips
- This **can** be frozen.

Making Time
Approximately 30–40 minutes

Makes
4 / 6 portions

Per Portion
20.1g carbs / 30.9g protein / 663 calories / 51.2g fat (*if 4 portions*)
13.4g carbs / 20.6g protein / 442 calories / 34.1g fat (*if 6 portions*)

INGREDIENTS

The Base Recipe
- 1 batch salsa (page 52)

The Rest of the Ingredients
All the vegetables, and the chorizo and the cheese, need to be chunky chopped.
- 400g butternut squash or swede (macros are based on swede)
- 400g courgette
- 400g peppers
- 120g leeks
- 200g chorizo
- 200g mature cheddar cheese
- 2 teaspoons paprika
- 2 teaspoons garlic puree or 4 garlic cloves, finely chopped
- 30g olive oil
- Salt and pepper (season to taste)

The Toppings
- 100g crème fraiche
- 1 heaped tablespoon fresh chives, finely chopped

METHOD

The Base Recipe
1. Make the salsa (page 52)

The Rest of the Ingredients
2. Heat the oven to 190°C or the Ninja to 180°C.
3. Apart from the crème fraiche, chives and the salsa, put all the other ingredients into an ovenproof dish and mix well.
4. Bake for about 30 minutes or pan fry for about 15–20 minutes or until all the vegetables are cooked.
5. Once the vegetables are cooked, stir in the salsa.
6. This is lovely hot or cold.

The Toppings
7. Add the crème fraiche and finely chopped chives (the crème fraiche can be stirred through or dolloped on top, and then sprinkle with the chives). Enjoy! ❤

Chicken and Parmesan

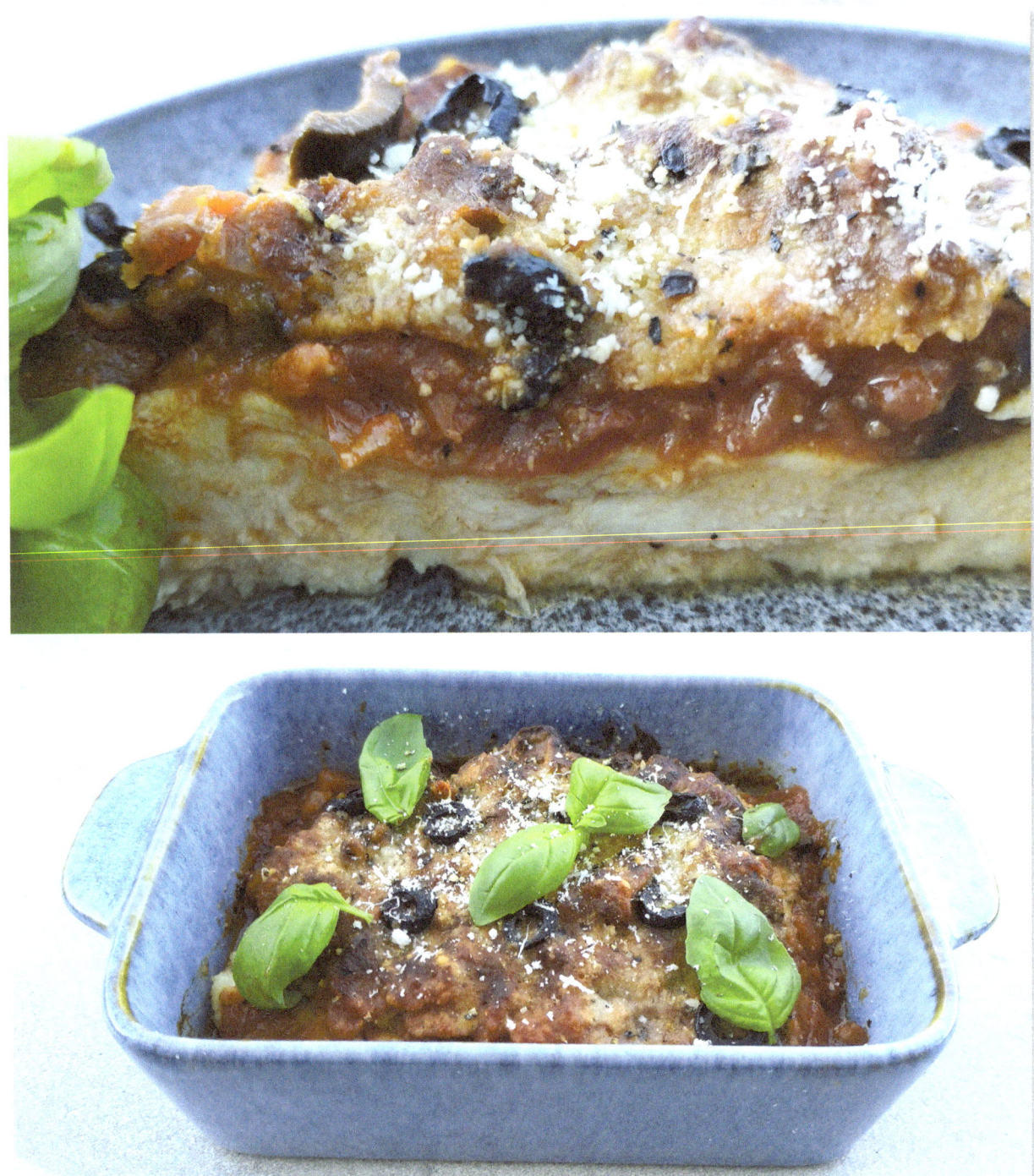

This is such a quick dish to prepare. Just choose your favourite vegetables, salad or even the rainbow rice recipe on page 42 to serve with it.

Equipment
- Ovenproof dish

Top Tips
- This **can** be frozen.

Making Time
Approximately 45 minutes

Makes
4 portions

Per Portion
4.9g carbs / 43.4g protein / 312 calories / 12.9g fat

INGREDIENTS

The Base Recipe
- 1 batch salsa (page 52)

The Rest of the Ingredients
- 600g chicken breast, flattened (you could use a rolling pin for this or a meat tenderiser) Top tip: pop some cling film on top before you do this.
- 60g parmesan, grated
- Salt and pepper

METHOD

The Base Recipe
1. Make the salsa (page 52)

The Rest of the Ingredients
2. Heat the oven to 180°C or the Ninja to 170°C.
3. Season the tenderised chicken breasts with salt and pepper.
4. Pop into a greased ovenproof dish, side by side, or I portioned mine into individual oven dishes.

NOTE TO CHEF If you are eating this whole dish immediately, please ignore this note! If you are eating this dish later, or if you are planning on freezing it, then wait for the salsa to cool before putting it on top of the chicken. This is to protect you from any unnecessary harmful bacteria.

5. Cover the chicken completely with your salsa.
6. Sprinkle with parmesan. I like to put a little ground pepper on top too.
7. Bake for approximately 20–30 minutes until chicken is completely cooked. Enjoy! ♥

Salmon and Green Vegetable Parcel

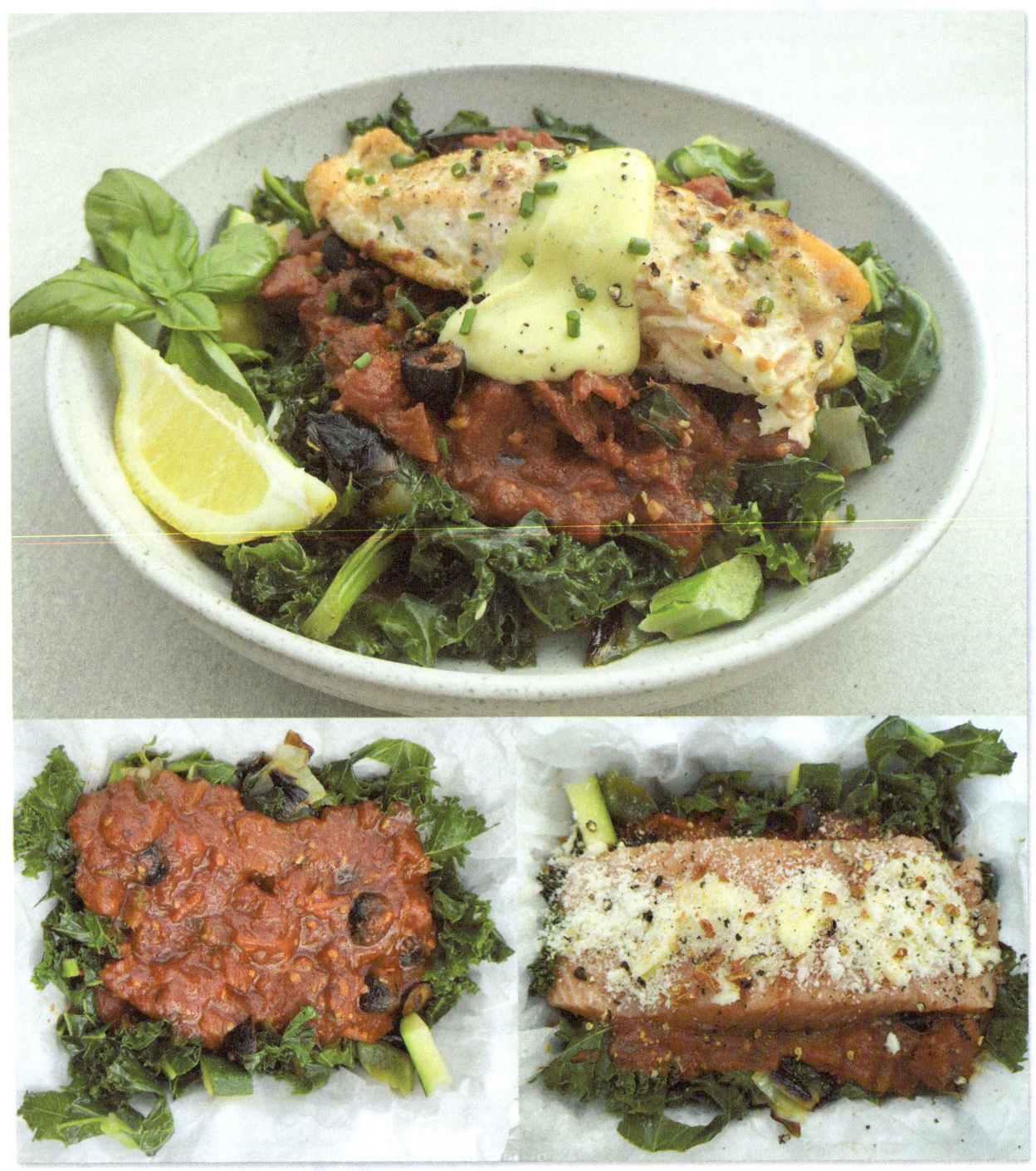

This is a superb recipe; everything you need for one meal, all wrapped up into one convenient parcel.

Equipment
- Greaseproof paper
- Kitchen string

Top Tips
- This **can** be frozen.

Making Time Approximately 45 minutes

Makes
4 portions

Per Portion
12.8g carbs / 42.7g protein / 639 calories / 46.2g fat

INGREDIENTS

The Base Recipe
- 1 batch salsa (page 52)

The Rest of the Ingredients
- 60g butter (40g to fry the leeks and 20g to spread on top the salmon)

All the green vegetables need to be chunky chopped.
- 200g leeks
- 200g broccoli
- 200g green beans
- 200g courgettes
- 200g curly kale
- 600g salmon fillet (or any fish of your choice)
- 40g Parmesan
- 5g chilli flakes
- Salt and pepper

METHOD

The Base Recipe
1. Make the salsa (page 52)

The Rest of the Ingredients
2. Heat the oven to 180°C or the Ninja to 170°C.
3. Meanwhile, lightly fry the leeks in the butter (40 g) for about 5 minutes or until translucent but not browned.
4. Now add all the other green vegetables and fry for another 5 minutes or until softened. Alternatively steam for 8–10 minutes and then remove from heat and stir butter through and season.
5. While this is cooking, cut up four sheets of greaseproof paper into large enough pieces to wrap around the vegetables, salsa and salmon, to create parcels.
6. Lay the greaseproof sheets down on the worktop and then divide all the partially cooked green vegetables in the centre of these four sheets.
7. Cover all the green vegetables evenly with the cooked salsa.

NOTE TO CHEF If you are cooking this whole dish immediately, please ignore this note! If you are eating this dish later, or if you're planning on freezing it, then wait for the salsa and cooked vegetables to cool before putting the fish on top. This is to protect you from any unnecessary harmful bacteria.

8. Now pop the salmon fillet on top.
9. Spread the remaining butter on each fillet (5g per fillet).
10. Sprinkle 10g Parmesan over each buttered fillet.
11. Finally, season the salmon well with salt and pepper and chilli flakes.
12. Create a parcel using your greaseproof paper and tie with the string. If you're freezing this dish, I would also wrap it in foil.
13. Bake for approximately 25–30 minutes or until the salmon is completely cooked. Enjoy! ♥

Tortilla Chips and Three Mexican Dips

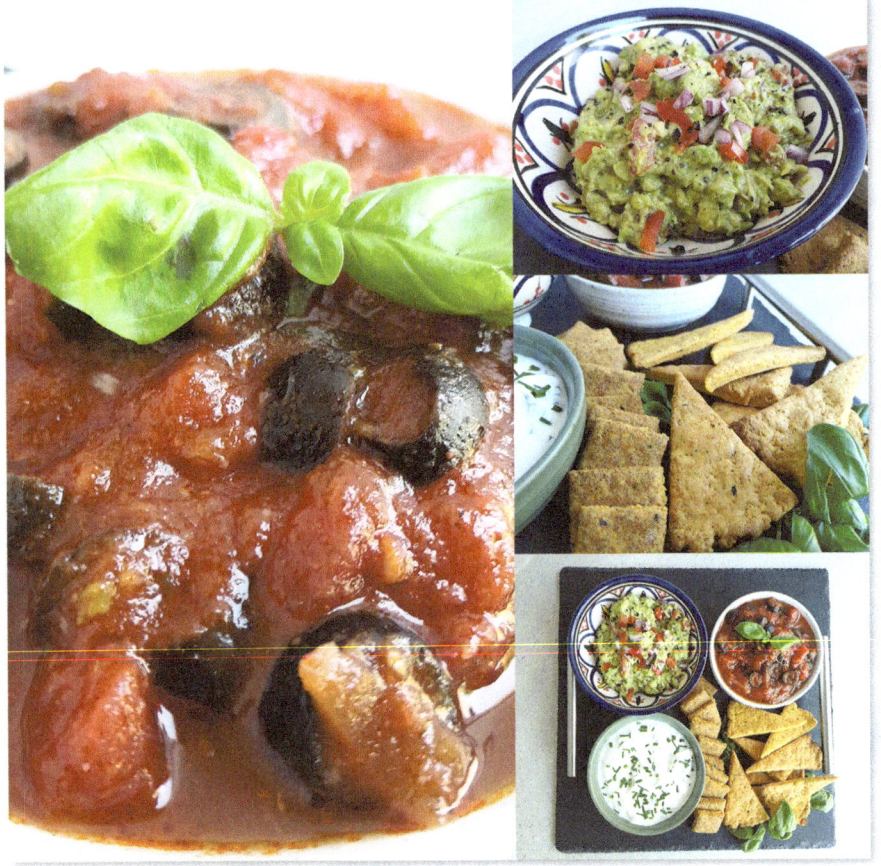

I really enjoyed creating this dish, as it says to me, 'Saturday night in, let's-watch-a movie type of food!' You also have two tortilla recipes to choose from. I couldn't decide which was my favourite, so you decide!

Equipment
- Lots of lovely serving bowls
- Tortilla press (If you like the idea of making wraps regularly, then you'll love the tortilla press gadget. It will make life a whole lot easier. Check out the pictures on page xv)

Top Tips
- This **cannot** be frozen, apart from the salsa.

Making Time
Approximately 45 minutes

Makes 4 / 6 portions

Per Portion
These are the whole-recipe macros, which includes the salsa, guacamole, sour cream and lupin tortilla if using **chips no.1:**
13.2g carbs / 21g protein / 439 calories / 32g fat (*if 4 portions*)
8.8g carbs / 14g protein / 293 calories / 21.4g fat (*if 6 portions*)
These are the whole-recipe macros, which include the salsa, guacamole, sour cream and lupin tortilla if using **chips no.2:**
11.5g carbs / 15.3g protein / 400 calories / 30.7g fat (*if 4 portions*)
7.7g carbs / 10.2g protein / 267 calories / 20.5g fat (*if 6 portions*)

One Salsa Four Ways

Salsa whole recipe contains:
18.9g carbs / 7.7g protein / 362 calories / 27.2g fat
Sour cream whole recipe contains:
4.4g carbs / 3g protein / 231 calories / 22.2g fat
Guacamole whole recipe contains:
7.2g carbs / 5g protein / 443 calories / 44g fat

Lupin tortilla chips no.1 whole recipe contains:
22.2g carbs / 69.7g protein / 742 calories / 35.2g fat
Lupin tortilla chips no.2 whole recipe contains:
15.2g carbs / 46.7g protein / 585 calories / 29.8g fat

INGREDIENTS

The Base Recipe
- 1 batch salsa (page 52)

The Rest of the Ingredients
Two different options for the chips…

Tortilla chips no.1 (triangles)
- 150g lupin flour
- ½ teaspoon baking powder
- ½ teaspoon xanthan gum
- ½ teaspoon salt
- ¼ teaspoon freshly ground pepper
- 1 teaspoon paprika or ½ teaspoon garlic powder
- 20g olive oil
- 100g warm water

Tortilla chips no.2 (squares)
- 100g lupin flour
- ½ teaspoon baking powder
- 20g psyllium husk
- ½ teaspoon salt
- ¼ teaspoon freshly ground pepper
- 1 teaspoon paprika or ½ teaspoon garlic powder
- 20g olive oil
- 100g warm water

The Guacamole
- 3–4 small avocados (once skinned and stoned, this is approximately 250 g)
- 40g red peppers, very finely chopped
- 10g red onion, finely chopped
- Zest of 1 lime
- 10ml freshly squeezed lime juice
- ½ teaspoon garlic puree or 1 garlic clove, finely chopped
- ¼ teaspoon Kashmiri chilli (I chose this chilli because of its gentle warmth, but any chilli powder is okay to use)
- ½ teaspoon salt
- ¼ teaspoon freshly ground black pepper

The Optional Extra
- 1 tablespoon coriander, finely chopped

The Sour Cream
- 120g sour cream
- 5g or approximately 2–3 teaspoons fresh chives, finely chopped

METHOD

The Base Recipe
1. Make the salsa (page 52)

The Tortilla Chips (choose your chip recipe!)
2. Heat the oven to 190°C or the Ninja to 180°C.
3. Add all the dry ingredients to a bowl and mix.
4. Add the oil and warm water and mix well.
5. I used a tortilla press for this bit, which I highly recommend. If not, roll into four equal balls and roll out between two pieces of greaseproof paper, until they are about 1–2 mm thick.
6. Score into triangular or square shapes.
7. Cook on the greaseproof paper for about 12–15 minutes. Cook until a little brown at the edges, but that's it!

The Guacamole
8. Mash up all the avocado flesh in a bowl.
9. Add all the other ingredients and mix well.

The Sour Cream and Chives
10. Add the sour cream and chives to a bowl and mix well. Enjoy! ♥

One Soup
Four Ways

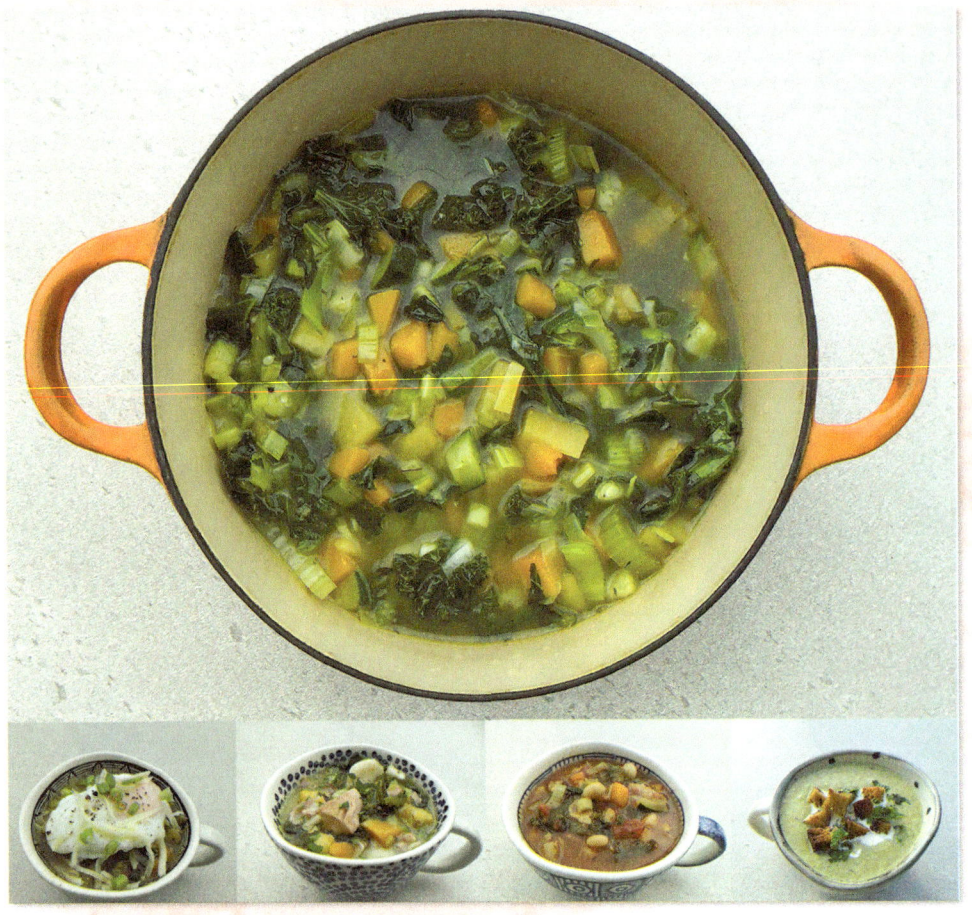

For this recipe, one soup base leads to four totally different, yet delicious, soups. This base recipe is super delicious on its own, but you'll love the soups that spin off from it.

Equipment
- Large non-stick saucepan

Top Tips
- This **can** be frozen.

Making Time
Approximately 30–40 minutes

Four Ways
Chicken and egg (page 64); Chowder (page 66); Minestrone (page 68); Vegetable smooth and creamy (page 70)

Makes
4 / 6 portions

Per Portion
8.8g carbs / 3.9g protein / 178 calories / 14.8g fat
(*if 4 portions*)
5.9g carbs / 2.6g protein / 119 calories / 9.9g fat
(*if 6 portions*)

INGREDIENTS
All the vegetables are to be small roughly chopped.
- 300g swede
- 30g olive oil
- 30g butter (to keep this dairy free, just use 30g olive oil or coconut oil)
- 200g winter greens (I use curly kale)
- 100g courgette
- 100g leek
- 50g celery
- ½ teaspoon garlic puree or 2 garlic cloves, finely chopped
- ½ teaspoon curry powder
- ½ teaspoon dried thyme
- 1 litre boiling water
- 2 vegetable stock cubes
- Salt and pepper to taste (I add ½ teaspoon salt and ¼ teaspoon freshly ground pepper)

METHOD
If you'd like to speed up the cooking time of this dish, prep your swede first and either steam it or boil it for about 10–15 minutes or pop it into a microwave bowl with a little water and cook on full power for about 5 minutes.

1. Put the oil and butter into a large non-stick saucepan. Once sizzling, add all your vegetables and fry for about 5 minutes. This is not to brown; it's purely to bring out their flavour.
2. Now add the garlic, curry powder and thyme. Stir through and cook for 2 minutes.
3. Add the boiling water, stock cubes and seasoning and stir.

   a. **If you're making the chicken and egg, add the chicken, mushrooms, ginger and liquid aminos now (page 64).**
   b. **If you're making the chowder, add the fish, bacon and cayenne pepper now (page 66).**
   c. **If you're making the minestrone, add the bacon now (page 68).**
   d. **If you're making the vegetable smooth and creamy, follow to the end of this recipe and then flip back to the vegetable smooth and creamy (page 70).**

4. Give whichever lovely soup you're making a good stir. Bring to a boil and turn down to a medium simmer (halfway between low and medium).
5. Cook until all the vegetables (and meats, if any) are cooked (about 30 minutes).
6. And that's the base done, or you're partway through one of the other recipes. It's a really nice soup on its own, but if you're partway through one of the other recipes, now flip back to whichever one you're making. Enjoy! ❤

Chicken and Egg Soup

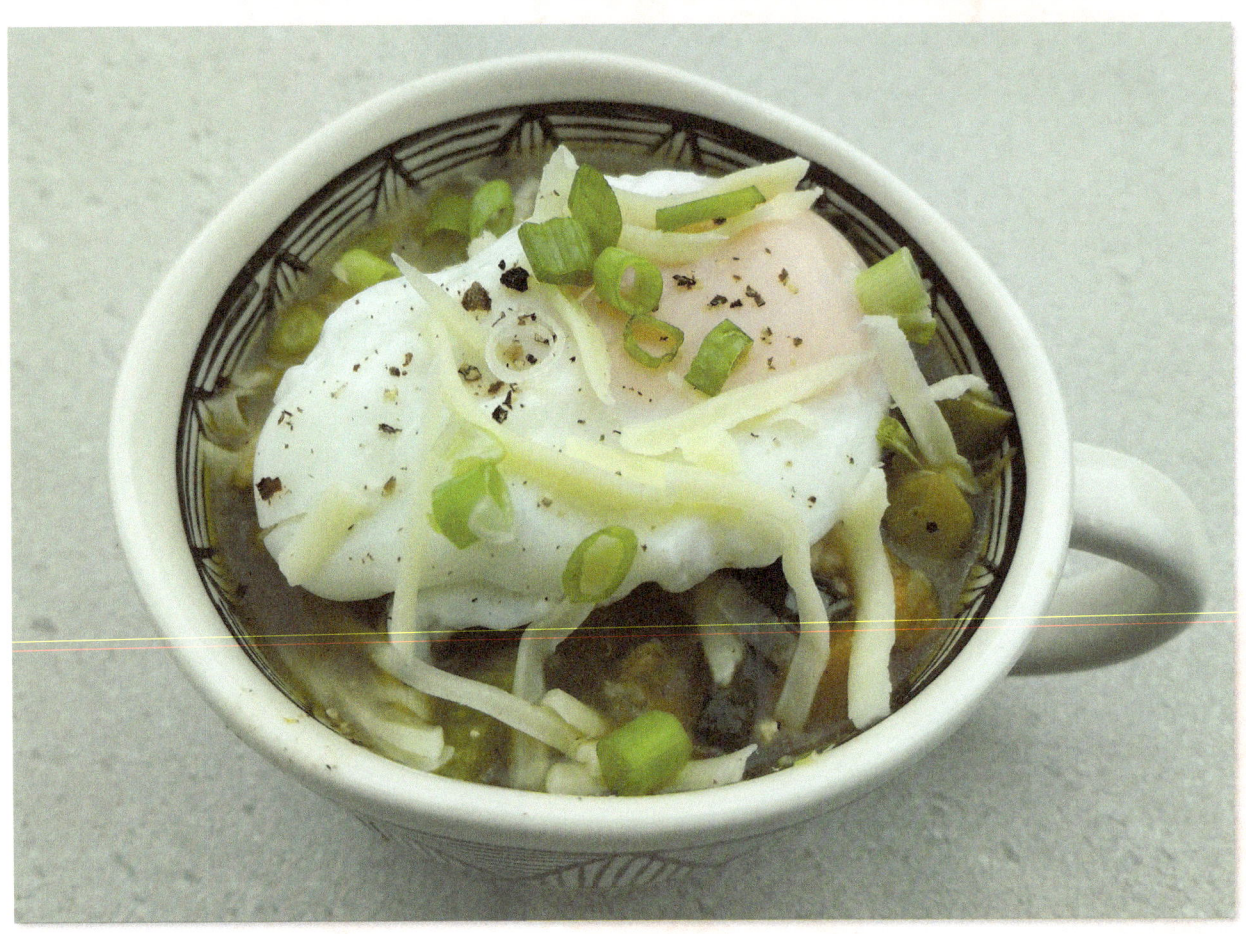

Adding poached egg before serving finishes off a really delicious soup.

One Soup **Four Ways**

Equipment
- Large non-stick saucepan
- Saucepan for making the poached eggs

Top Tips
- This **cannot** be frozen unless you add the poached eggs fresh, after defrosting.

Making Time
Approximately 45 minutes

Makes
4 / 6 portions

Per Portion
10.5g carbs / 36.6g protein / 418 calories / 26.2g fat
(*if 4 portions, each with 1 egg*)
7g carbs / 26.8g protein / 304 calories / 19.2g fat
(*if 6 portions, each with 1 egg*)

INGREDIENTS

The Base Recipe
- 1 batch soup (page 62)

The Rest of the Ingredients
- 300g chicken, chunky chopped
- 75g mushrooms, chunky chopped
- 1½ teaspoons ginger puree or 2½ teaspoons fresh ginger, finely chopped.
- 25ml liquid aminos (this is a soy sauce replacement)
- 4–6 large eggs (depending on whether it's a 4 – or 6-portion soup)
- 100g fresh or ready-grated mozzarella
- 75g spring onions, chunky chopped
- Extra seasoning, if required

METHOD

The Base Recipe
1. Make the soup (page 62).
   ** Watch out for Step 3 in the base recipe, where you add the chicken, mushrooms, ginger and liquid aminos.

The Rest of the Ingredients
2. For the poached eggs, bring a saucepan, about 3 cm deep with water, to a boil. Crack your eggs directly into the water and boil for about 3 minutes.
3. Dish up your soup and top it with the poached egg.
4. Sprinkle the spring onion and the mozzarella over each bowl. Enjoy! ♥

Chowder

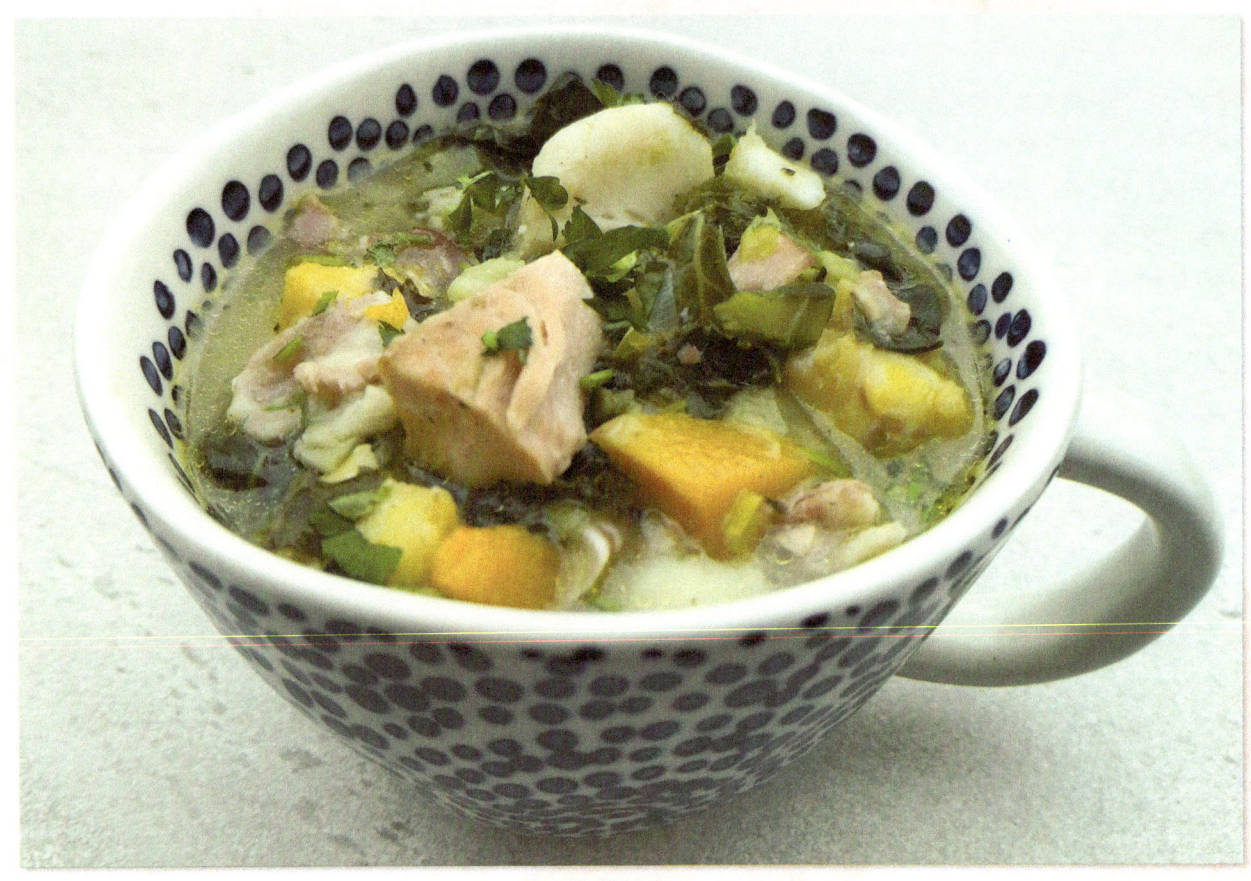

This soup is my take on a really nice fishy soup. It's lovely.

Equipment
- Large non-stick saucepan

Top Tips
- This **can** be frozen.

Making Time
Approximately 45 minutes

Makes
4 / 6 portions

Per Portion
15.2g carbs / 35.3g protein / 433 calories / 26.5g fat (*if 4 portions*)
10.1g carbs / 23.5g protein / 289 calories / 17.7g fat (*if 6 portions*)

INGREDIENTS

The Base Recipe
- 1 batch soup (page 62)

The Rest of the Ingredients
- 600g fish mix
- 100g bacon, small roughly chopped
- Pinch cayenne pepper
- 200ml coconut milk
- 30g parsley, finely chopped (**save 5g for sprinkling as a garnish over each bowl**)

METHOD

The Base Recipe
1. Make the soup (page 62).
   **Watch out for Step 3 in the base recipe, where you add the fish, bacon and cayenne pepper.

The Rest of the Ingredients
2. Once you have followed the base recipe, add the final ingredients: coconut milk and parsley (25 g).
3. Heat through and serve.
4. Sprinkle the remaining parsley (5 g). Enjoy! ♥

Minestrone Soup

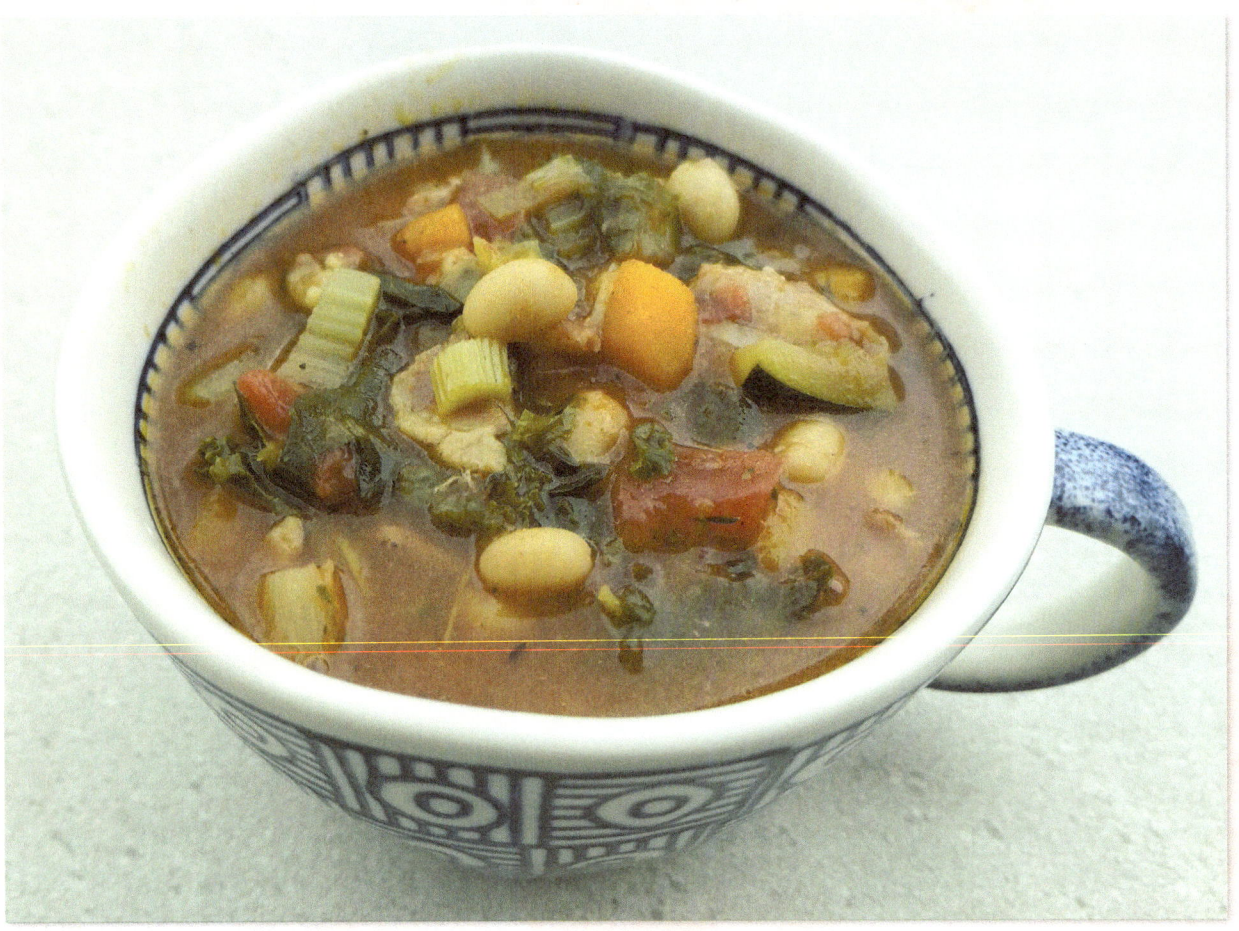

This soup is a memory soup. My dad always made this for us when we were younger. After he died, I kept a tub in the freezer for years. So this is my low-carb version of a lovely memory. Hope you love it too! Normally, this soup would have pasta in it, but this recipe doesn't. It would also have a selection of beans in it. For my own personal soup satisfaction, I have kept the beans in, and I have included the macros for that, but I have also included the macros for the recipe without the beans (quite a difference, but not nearly as nice in my opinion).

Equipment
- Large non-stick saucepan

Top Tips
- This **can** be frozen.

Making Time
Approximately 45 minutes

Makes
4 / 6 portions

Per Portion
With haricot beans:
20.2g carbs / 14.1g protein / 319 calories / 20.1g fat (*if 4 portions*)
13.5g carbs / 9.4g protein / 212 calories / 13.4g fat (*if 6 portions*)

Without haricot beans:
14.5g carbs / 11.9g protein / 280 calories / 19.7g Fat (*if 4 portions*)
9.7g carbs / 7.9g protein / 186 calories / 13.2g Fat (*if 6 portions*)

For the whole recipe:
80.8g carbs / 56.3g protein / 1274 calories / 80.5g fat (*with haricot beans*)
58g carbs / 47.4g protein / 1118 calories / 79g fat (*without haricot beans*)

INGREDIENTS
The Base Recipe
- 1 batch soup (page 62)

The Rest of the Ingredients
- 150g bacon, chunky chopped
- 200g tinned tomatoes
- 150g haricot beans (these can be omitted — see the description above)
- 100g tomato puree
- 1 teaspoon dried oregano or mixed herbs
- ½ teaspoon paprika
- 250ml boiling water (if you feel you need it)
- Extra seasoning (if required)

METHOD
The Base Recipe
1. Make the soup (page 62).
   ** Watch out for Step 3 in the base recipe, where you add the bacon.

The Rest of the Ingredients
2. Once you have followed the base recipe, add all the other ingredients and stir through.
3. Bring to temperature. Enjoy! ♥

Vegetable Smooth and Creamy Soup

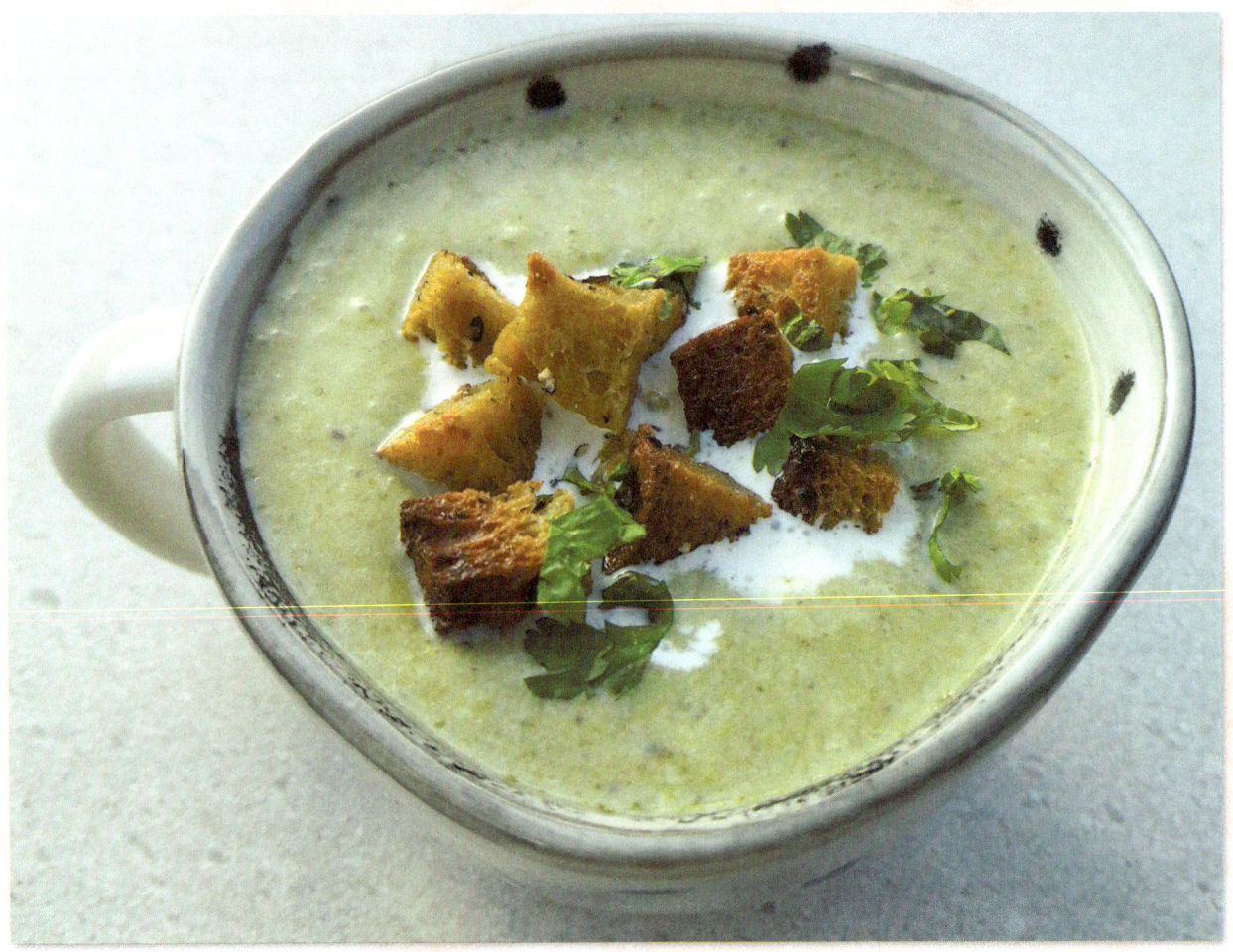

This soup has only one extra ingredient which makes all the difference when making it a transformation from the base soup. To make this into more of a meal, serve with a protein of your choice. For me, it's got to be a poached egg.

Equipment
- Large non-stick saucepan
- Hand blender or liquidiser

Top Tips
- For the perfect super-smooth soup, all the vegetables need to be really well cooked.
- This **can** be frozen (without the egg).

Making Time
Approximately 40 minutes

Makes
4 / 6 portions

Per Portion
9.5g carbs / 4.5g protein / 382 calories / 36.9g fat (*if 4 portions*)
6.3g carbs / 3g protein / 255 calories / 24.6g fat (*if 6 portions*)

INGREDIENTS
The Base Recipe
- 1 batch soup (page 62)

The Rest of the Ingredients
- 175ml double cream or coconut milk

METHOD
The Base Recipe
- Make the soup (page 62)

The Rest of the Ingredients
1. Once you have followed the base recipe, add the double cream or coconut milk and blitz until super smooth. Enjoy! ♥

One Yorkshire Pudding Four Ways

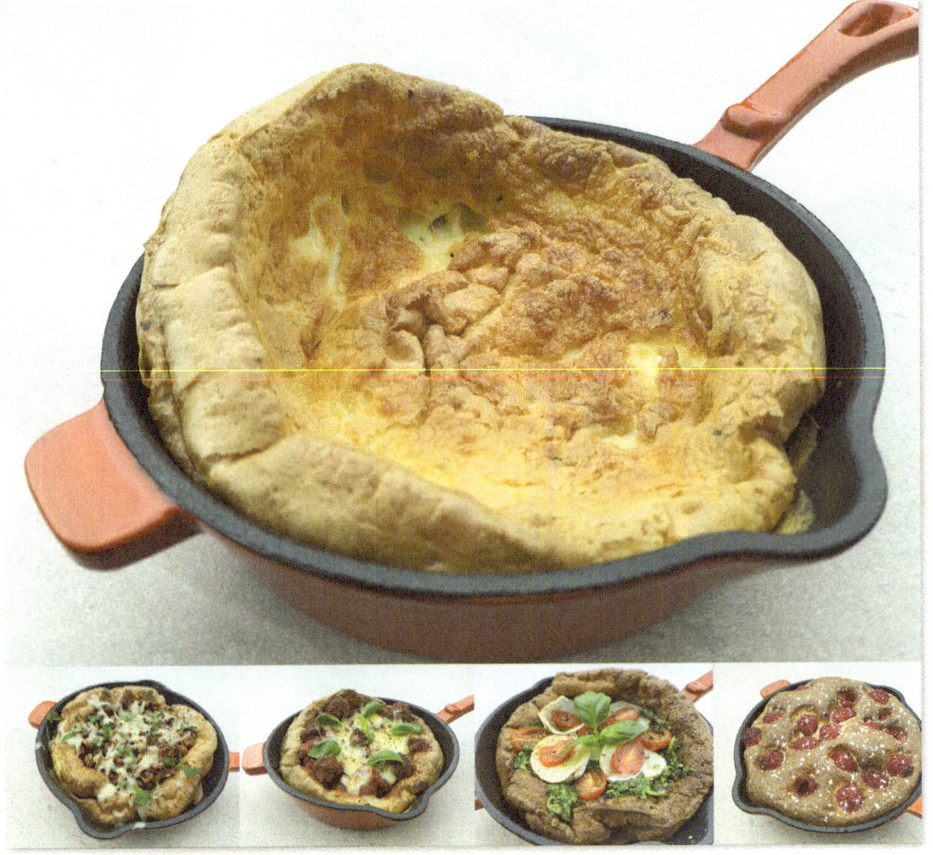

I love the idea of a Yorkshire pudding with the meal contents safely packed into it, pizza style. I do hope you enjoy it as much as we do!

Of course, it also makes a great Yorkshire pudding on its own.

Once you have the toppings on, depending on how much sauce there is, the bottom may go a little soggy. This does not take away from the recipe being a success and super tasty.

Equipment
- 2 x non-stick baking tins, approximately 15–17cms in diameter, or 1 larger tin (or if you want it as a light snack, 4 individual tins)
- Bullet or a hand blender

Top Tips
- The ratios in this recipe work really well. Make sure that the cream/milk mix comes in at the same weight as the eggs. For example if the egg weight comes in at 120 g, change the liquids to 120g too. I prefer a higher content of cream to milk, so in this case I would have 75g cream and 45g milk. Whatever your egg weight is, times that by 0.15 for your arrowroot quantity (e.g. 120 x 0.15 = arrowroot 18 g).
- This **can** be frozen.

Making Time
Approximately 20 minutes

Makes
2 / 4 portions

Per Portion
This dish is designed for two portions, but if you'd like it as a snack, I've included the macros for four portions as well:
10.3g carbs / 8.8g protein / 381 calories / 33.7g fat *(if 2 portions)*
5.1g carbs / 4.4g protein / 190 calories / 16.9g fat *(if 4 portions)*

Four Ways
Lamb and leek (page 74) Meatballs in a tomato sauce (page 76); Pesto and goat's cheese (page 78); Raspberry popover (page 80)

INGREDIENTS
- 15g lard or coconut oil if you're making the raspberry popover on (page 80)
- 80g double cream
- 50g milk of your choice (I like to use full fat lactose free milk)
- 20g arrowroot powder
- 2 large eggs (approximately 130 g)
- Seasoning (I add ¼ teaspoon salt and a good grind of pepper (**no seasoning if you're making the raspberry popover** (page 80)

METHOD
1. Heat the oven to 210°C or the Ninja to 200°C.
2. Add the lard or coconut oil to a baking tin and pop in the oven for about 5 minutes or until it's sizzling hot.
3. Meanwhile, add the remaining ingredients to a bowl or blender and whisk up until smooth.
4. Back to the oven. After about 5 minutes, remove the baking tin from the oven carefully. Check that the oil is hot enough by dropping a tiny amount of the mix into the oil. The oil should bubble around the mix. If not, return the tin to the oven for a few more minutes.
5. When the oil is ready, pour the mix into the tin or tins.
6. Bake for approximately 15–20 minutes or until golden and crispy.
7. Enjoy as a Yorkshire pudding, or move on to one of the other four delicious recipes. Enjoy! ♥

Lamb and Leek

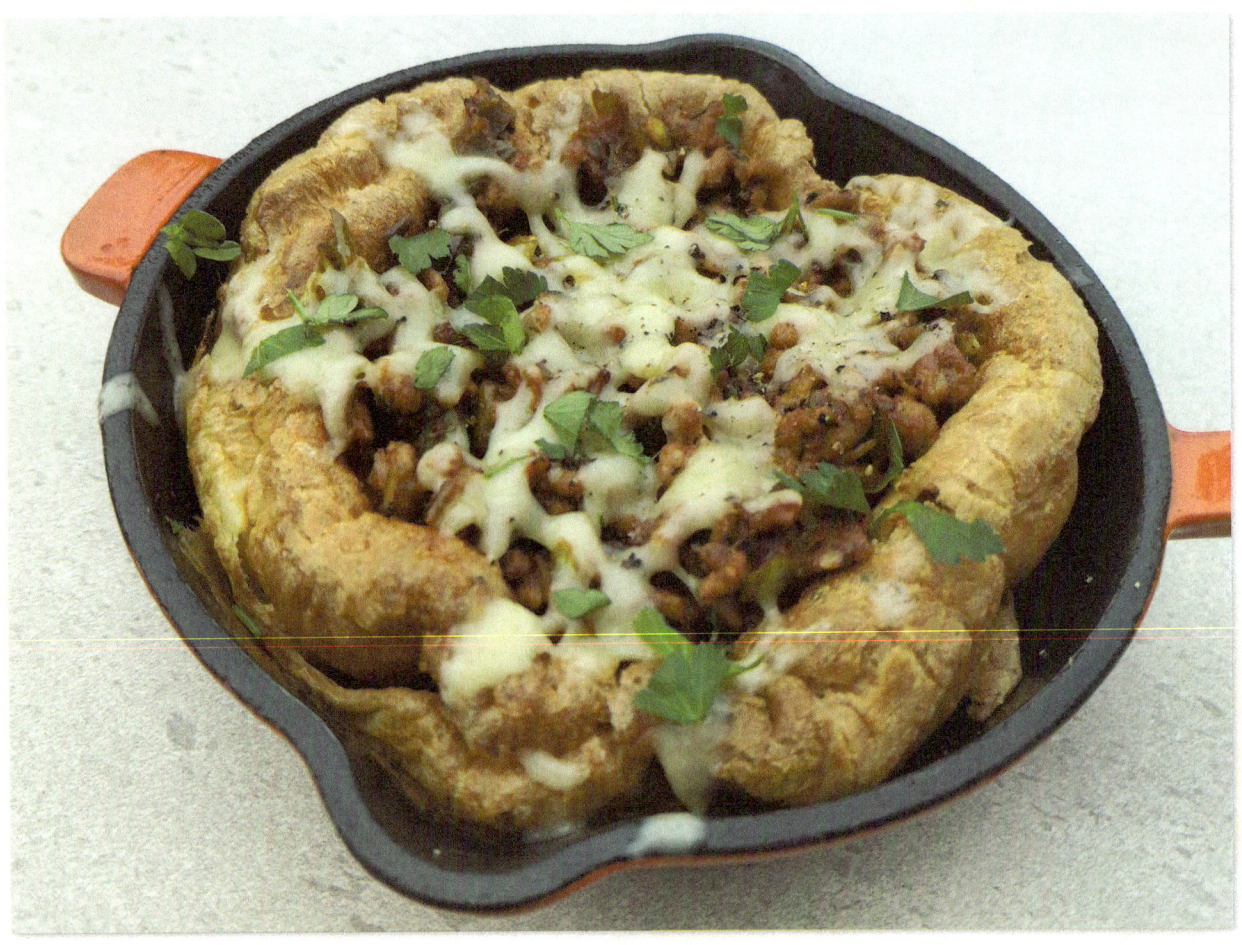

You know what I like about this particular Yorkshire pudding dish, apart from being super tasty, it's also super quick to make.

Equipment
- 2 x non-stick baking tins approximately 15–17 cm in diameter or 1 larger tin
- A bullet or hand blender
- Non-stick frying pan

Top Tips
- You can swap the lamb mince for beef, turkey or chicken mince. If you use turkey or chicken mince, you may need a little more seasoning in the topping.
- This **can** be frozen.

Making Time
Approximately 25 minutes

Makes
2 / 4 portions

Per Portion
This dish is designed for two portions, but if you'd like it as a snack, I've included the macros for two portions as well:
14.2g carbs / 30.8g protein / 680 calories / 55.7g fat (*if 2 portions*)
7.1g carbs / 15.4g protein / 340 calories / 27.9g fat (*if 4 portions*)

INGREDIENTS
The Base Recipe
- 1 batch Yorkshire pudding (page 72)

The Topping
- 10g olive oil
- 50g leeks, finely chopped
- 200g lamb mince
- 30g courgette, grated
- 30g tomato puree
- ¼ teaspoon garlic puree or 1 small garlic clove finely chopped
- ¼ teaspoon curry powder
- Salt and pepper (I add ¼ teaspoon salt and a good grind of freshly ground black pepper)
- 30g mature cheddar grated

METHOD
The Base Recipe
1. Make the Yorkshire pudding (page 72).
2. While the Yorkshire Pudding base is cooking, move on to the topping.

The Topping
3. Add the olive oil to the frying pan and heat it up until it's sizzling. Then turn the temperature down to a medium temperature, add the leeks and fry for about 3–5 minutes or until translucent but not browned.
4. Add the lamb mince and courgette and fry for a further 5 minutes.
5. Now add all the other topping ingredients to the pan (**apart from the cheese**).
6. Add a little boiling water to the pan to give it a small sauce.
7. When your base is cooked, spread the lamb topping over the Yorkshire pudding.
8. Sprinkle over the cheese and pop back in the oven for about 5 minutes or until the cheese has melted. Enjoy! ♥

Meatballs in a Tomato Sauce

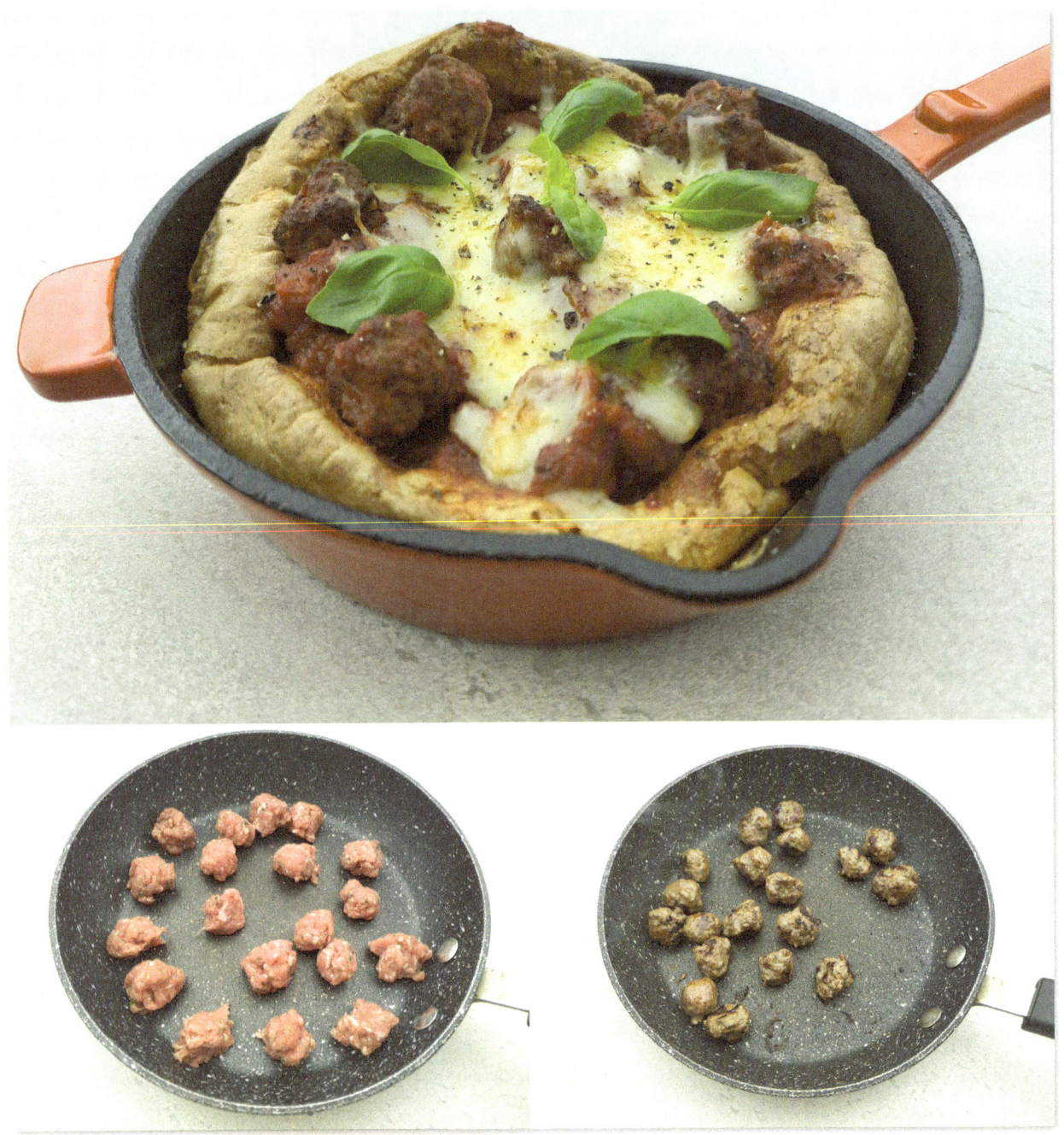

Apart from this being a delightful family pleaser, you'll also get to taste and use the tomato sauce recipe on page 104, which is a perfect condiment for any dish.

Equipment
- 2 x non-stick baking tins approximately 15–17 cms in diameter or 1 larger tin
- A bullet or hand blender
- Non-stick frying pan

Top Tips
- You can swap the beef mince for lamb, turkey or chicken mince. If you use turkey or chicken mince, you may need a little more seasoning in the topping.
- This **can** be frozen.

Making Time
Approximately 25 minutes

Makes
2 / 4 portions

Per Portion
This dish is designed for two portions, but if you'd like it as a snack, I've included the macros for four portions as well:
17.8g carbs / 37.3g protein / 674 calories / 50.3g fat *(if 2 portions)*
8.9g carbs / 18.6g protein / 337 calories / 25.1g fat *(if 4 portions)*

INGREDIENTS

The Base Recipe
- 1 batch Yorkshire Pudding (page 72)

The Meatballs
- 200g beef mince
- ½ teaspoon dried oregano or mixed herbs
- Salt and pepper (I add ¼ teaspoon salt and a good grind of freshly ground black pepper)

Tomato Sauce
- ½ batch of tomato sauce (page 104) (I recommend you make the whole recipe, as I'm sure you'll find many other uses for it.)

Cheese Topping
- 40g mature cheddar, grated

Optional Extra
- A sprinkling of basil leaves after the dish comes out of the oven

METHOD

The Base Recipe
1. Make the Yorkshire pudding (page 72).
2. While the Yorkshire pudding is cooking, move on to the topping.

The Meatballs
3. Put all the meatball ingredients into a bowl and mix well (I think hands are best).
4. If you have a non-stick frying pan, you don't need any oil, but if not, then give it a light coating of olive oil and heat the pan up.
5. Break the mince into little chunks and drop them into the frying pan, and fry them until they are almost cooked and holding together. This will take about 5–10 minutes.

The Tomato Sauce
6. Make the tomato sauce (page 104). (I recommend you make the whole recipe, as I'm sure you'll find many other uses for it.)
7. Now add the tomato sauce to your meatballs. Heat up until bubbling and simmer for about 10 minutes to reduce the sauce and finish off cooking the meatballs.

The Final Part of the Recipe
8. When your base is cooked, spread the meatball topping over the Yorkshire pudding.
9. Sprinkle over the cheese and pop back in the oven for about 3–5 minutes or until the cheese has melted.
10. Garnish with the basil if you are using. Enjoy! ♥

Pesto and Goat's Cheese

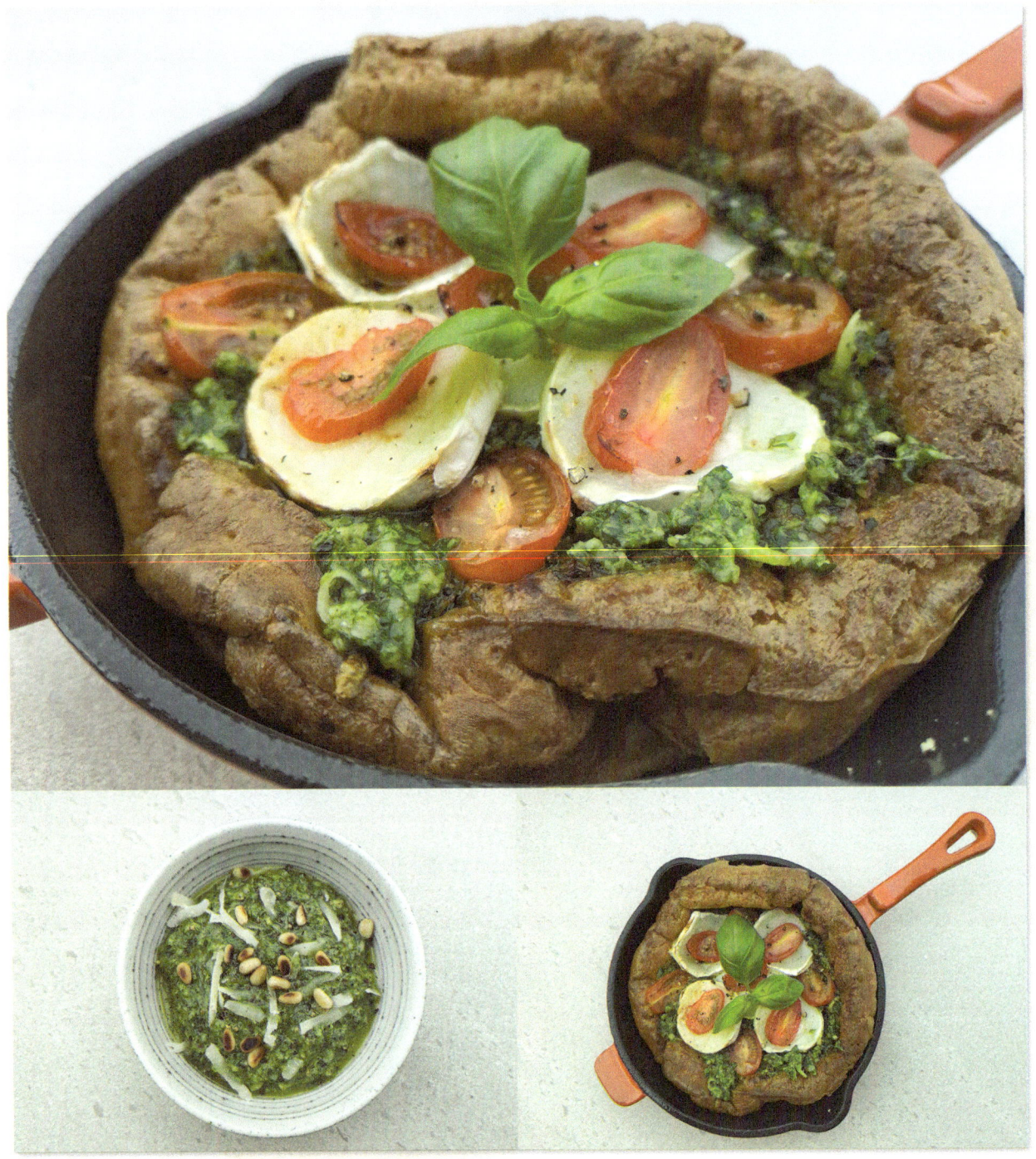

This makes a great starter or side dish, as well as a main meal. A great vegetarian alternative. You'll also have some leftover pesto for the fridge.

One Yorkshire Pudding **Four Ways**

Equipment
- 2 x non-stick baking tins approximately 15–17 cms in diameter or 1 larger tin
- A bullet or hand blender
- Small non-stick frying pan

Top Tips
- This **can** be frozen.

Making Time
Approximately 25 minutes

Makes
2 / 4 portions

Per Portion
This dish is designed for two portions, but if you'd like it as a snack, I've included the macros for four portions as well:

13g carbs / 25.4g protein / 808 calories / 72.7g fat (if 2 portions)

6.5g carbs / 12.7g protein / 404 calories / 36.4g fat (if 4 portions)

INGREDIENTS

The Base Recipe
- 1 batch Yorkshire pudding (page 72)

The Pesto
- ½ batch pesto (page 100)
  (I recommend you make the whole recipe, as I'm sure you'll find many other uses for it.)

The Rest of the Ingredients
- 120g goat's cheese, thinly sliced
- 50g cherry tomatoes, thinly sliced

METHOD

The Base Recipe
1. Make the Yorkshire pudding (page 72).
2. While the Yorkshire pudding is cooking, move on to the toppings.

The Pesto
3. Make half a batch of the pesto (page 100).
   (I recommend you make the whole recipe, as I'm sure you'll find many other uses for it.)

The Rest of the Ingredients and the Construction
4. Once you've made the Yordkshire pudding and the pesto, spread the pesto over the Yorkshire pudding.
5. Top with your sliced goat's cheese and cherry tomatoes.
6. Pop back in the oven for about 3–5 minutes. Enjoy! ♥

Raspberry Popover

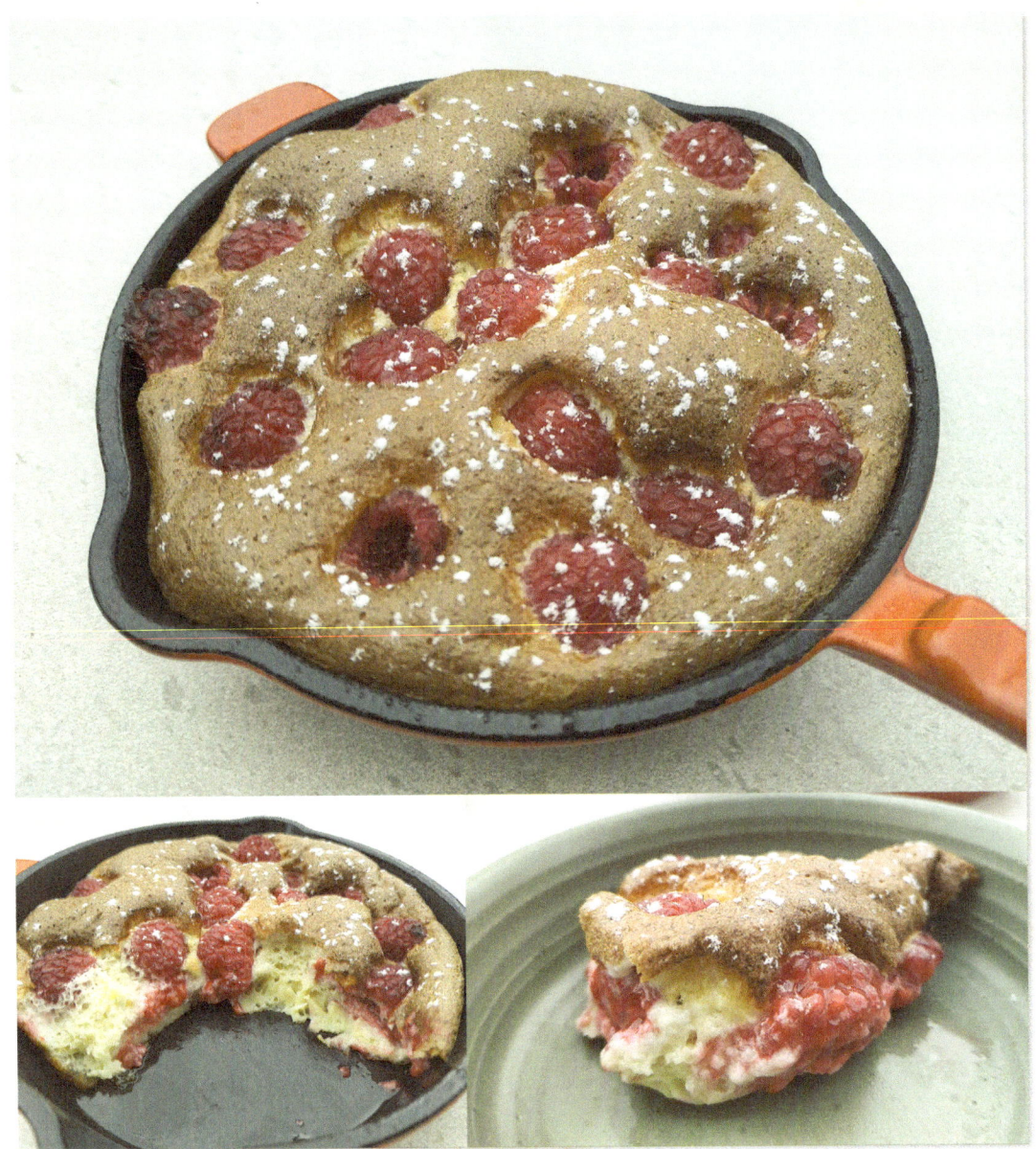

National Raspberry Popover Day on 3 May each year recognises a dish similar to Yorkshire pudding. The day is also referred to as National Raspberry Tart Day. My low-carb take on this is, in my opinion, is that it is just heavenly.

Popovers earn their name by their characteristic popping over the edge of the pan as they bake. The main ingredients in popovers are flour, eggs, milk, butter, salt and butter. The raspberries make the popovers sweeter, but you could swap them for another berry of your choice.

Equipment
- 2 x non-stick baking tins, approximately 15–17 cms in diameter, or 12 muffin tins, well oiled
- Bullet or hand blender

Top Tips
- This **cannot** be frozen.

Making Time
Approximately 20 minutes

Makes
12 portions

Per Portion
2.4g carbs / 1.6g protein / 67 calories / 5.7g fat

INGREDIENTS
The Base Recipe
- 1 batch Yorkshire pudding (page 72)
  (This is purely for the recipe ingredients, then pop back here for the instructions, as it's a completely different method for this recipe. Also, don't worry about weighing the eggs. Just use 2 large eggs and separate the whites from the egg yolks. Do not add the salt or pepper.)
- 30g Truvia sweetener icing
- 150g raspberries

The Final Ingredients
- 1 teaspoon Truvia icing sugar, just a little sprinkling for decoration

METHOD
The Base Recipe
1. Heat the oven to 180°C or the Ninja 170°C.
2. **This time use coconut oil for your baking tins and pop in the oven for approximately 5 minutes.**
3. Whisk up the egg whites to soft peaks.
4. In a separate bowl, whisk up the milk, cream, egg yolks, arrowroot and the sweetener.
5. Now carefully fold these ingredients into the egg whites until they are completely mixed. **You want to try to keep the air in as much as possible.**
6. Back to the tins in the oven. After 5 minutes, carefully remove the baking tin from the oven. Check that the oil is hot enough by dropping a tiny amount of the mix into the oil. The oil should bubble around the mix. If not, return the tin to the oven for a few more minutes.
7. When the oil is ready, pour the mix into the tins.
8. Sprinkle the raspberries over the top. They will sink in, but that's okay.
9. Cook for about 20–25 minutes in the oven or about 15–20 minutes in the Ninja.
10. These will grow and then shrink back. This will not take away from the fabulous taste.

The Final Ingredients

11. A little sprinkling of icing sugar and it looks even more fabulous. Enjoy! ♥

One Custard Tart Four Ways

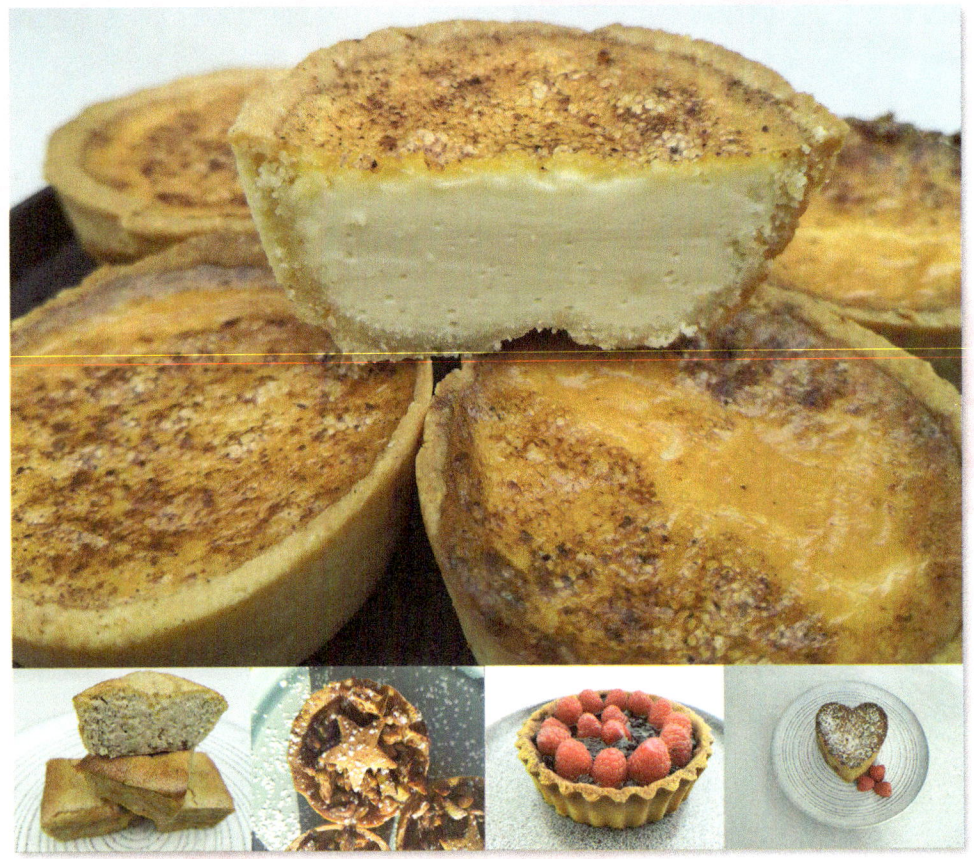

This is a simple custard tart recipe. There are so many recipes out there that it's hard to say which one works best. Some are all milk, some all cream, but this combination of cream and milk seems to work best for me. The other thing I like to do is add nutmeg to the custard and sprinkle on top.

These tarts don't rise that much, so make sure that you fill the pastry cups/large tin right to the top, as when it cools, it will shrink back a little.

Equipment
- A bullet, hand blender, food processor or a hand whisk
- Rolling pin
- 20 cms spring-based tin or a 12-portion muffin tray (You can either make this as one big tart or 12 individual portions.)

Top Tips
- This **can** be frozen.

Four Ways
Far breton (page 84); Festive apple crunch (page 86); Glazed fruit tart (page 88); Manchester tart (page 90)

Making Time
Approximately 40 minutes

Makes
12 portions

Per Portion
3.5g carbs / 6.2g protein / 219 calories / 19.8g fat

INGREDIENTS

The Pastry
- 150g ground almonds
- 75g butter, straight from the fridge and cut into small cubes
- 30g coconut flour
- 1 medium egg
- 2 teaspoons vanilla essence
- ½ teaspoon xanthan gum
- ⅛ teaspoon salt
- 30g Truvia sweetener (**optional sweetener for the pastry**)

The Custard Filling
**If you are making the glazed fruit tarts or the festive apple crunch, you only need half the quantity of custard filling, as this will be topped up with other ingredients.

- 4 medium eggs
- 175ml milk (I like to use full-fat lactose-free milk)
- 125ml double cream
- 30g Truvia sweetener
- 3 teaspoons vanilla essence
- ⅛ teaspoon salt
- ½ teaspoon nutmeg (**omit this for all the other recipes**)

METHOD

The Pastry
1. Heat the oven to 170°C or the Ninja to 160°C.
2. Add all the pastry ingredients to the food processor and blitz until it forms a lovely smooth dough ball. *Make sure the butter is straight from the fridge.*
3. If it's too sticky to roll, wait a few minutes, as the coconut will absorb the moisture, or add a little more coconut flour.
4. Roll out the pastry on a silicone rolling mat. If you need to, use a little coconut flour to stop it sticking.
5. Line a non-stick ovenproof dish or 12 cake tins with the pastry and gently press into the sides of the dish. It will possibly break as you're doing this. Don't worry; just use spare pieces of dough to patchwork it back together.
6. Pop in the Ninja for about 3 minutes or the oven for about 5–7 minutes on the middle shelf to par-bake.
7. If you are making the Manchester tart (page 90), pop back to that recipe and move on to **Step 2**.

The Custard Filling
8. Keep the oven at 170°C or the Ninja to 160°C.
9. Add all the custard ingredients, apart from half of the nutmeg, to a large mixing bowl or food processor and mix until smooth.
10. Pour the custard into the partially baked pastry cases or the large pastry and sprinkle the remaining nutmeg over the top of the custard.
11. If you're cooking 12 small tarts, these will cook a lot quicker than the large tart. Cook in the oven for approximately 20–25 minutes for 12 tarts and 30–45 minutes for one large tart, or in the Ninja for approximately 20 minutes for 12 tarts and 30–35 minutes for one large tart.
12. Allow to cool before removing from the tin. Enjoy! ♥

Far Breton

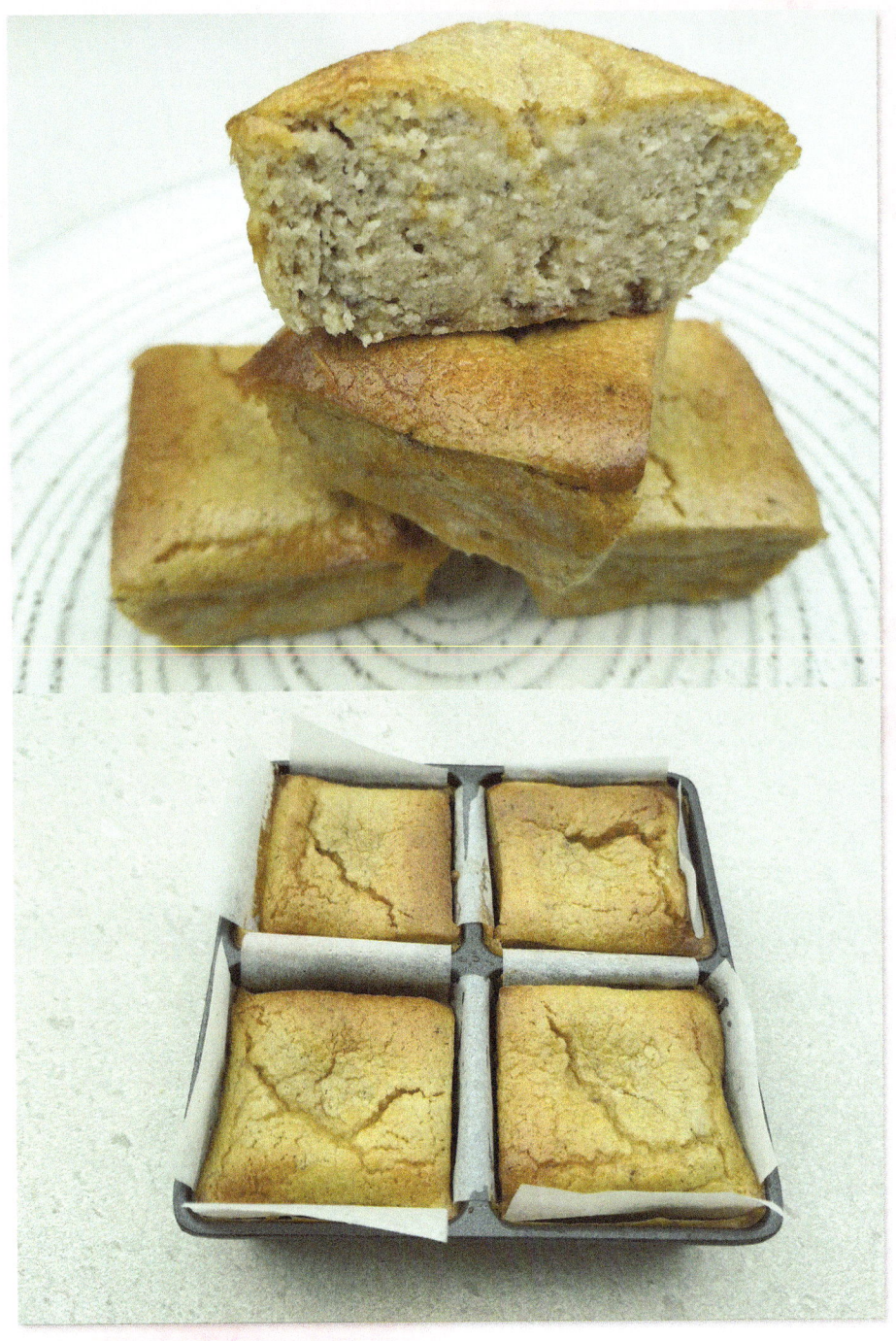

After a little research about this pudding, I thought what's not to like? A little dates and rum! This was a request by a friend for me to low carb, and this sat very comfortably in this custard tart section, but remember to ditch the pastry. This is meant to be a moist cake.

Equipment
- A bullet, hand blender, food processor or a hand whisk
- I used individual-portion brownie tins, but if you're using one large tin, approximately 16 cm x 16cm is perfect.

Top Tips
- This **can** be frozen.

Making Time
Approximately 30 minutes but allow an extra hour for soaking the dates

Makes
12 portions

Per Portion
5.2g carbs / 4.7g protein / 166 calories / 12.6g fat

INGREDIENTS

The Date Paste
- 50g dates, chopped really small
- 75g rum

The Base Recipe
- 1 batch custard tart (page 82) (Purely for the custard ingredients. Do **not** use the pastry ingredients or the **nutmeg**.)
- 120g ground almonds

METHOD

The Date Paste
1. Soak the rum and dates for an hour or so.
2. Whiz up to a fine puree.
3. Put this to one side while you work on the custard base.

The Base Recipe
4. In a large mixing bowl or food processor, add the custard ingredients and the ground almonds and mix until smooth.
5. Now pour the custard into the brownie tin.
6. Drizzle the date paste evenly across the custard.
7. Do not mix in, but with a cocktail stick or something similar, carefully and evenly swirl it in to create a marble effect.
8. Bake for approximately 30–45 minutes or until it's firm to touch.
9. Allow to cool. Enjoy! ♥

Festive Apple Crunch

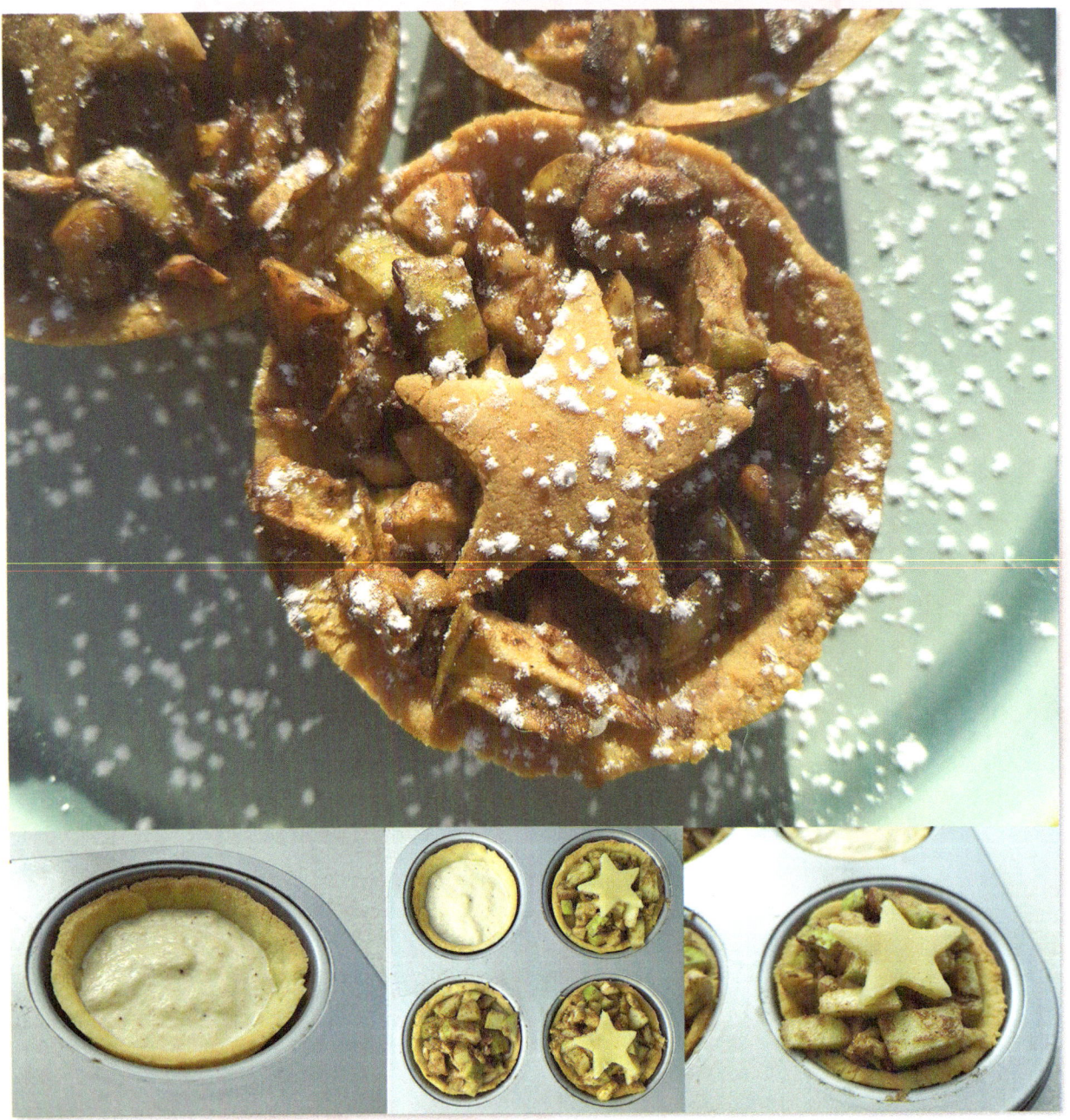

It's basically appple pie and custard. Adding the spices does give it a festive feel and nuts for that extra crunch.

Equipment
- A bullet, hand blender, food processor, or a hand whisk
- Large mixing bowl
- Rolling pin
- 20 cm spring-based tin or 12-portion muffin tray (You can either make this as one big tart or 12 individual portions.)

Top Tips
- As these were designed as a festive-style cake, I chose to decorate with stars, using leftover bits of pastry.
- This **can** be frozen.

Making Time
Approximately 30 minutes

Makes
12 portions

Per Portion
5.4g carbs / 7.1g protein / 262 calories / 23.3g fat

INGREDIENTS
The Base Recipe
- 1 batch custard tart (page 82) (**Please note that you will need to make up all of the pastry but only half of the custard filling, as this will be topped up with other ingredients**.)

The Rest of the Ingredients for the Topping
- 200g cooking apples, peeled, cored and small chunky chopped
- 100g mixed nuts, chunky chopped by hand (**do not blitz in the food processor**)
- 40g melted butter
- 1 teaspoon vanilla extract
- 1 teaspoon ground cinnamon or mixed spice
- 30g Truvia sweetener (for this recipe, I like to use the brown granulated)

METHOD
The Base Recipe
1. Make the custard tart (page 82), but stop when you've finished **Step 9** then jump back here.
2. Divide the custard between your pastry-lined and par-baked tins, half filling each pastry base case.

The Rest of the Ingredients for the Topping
3. Add all your topping ingredients to a large bowl and mix well.
4. Evenly spread across your uncooked custard.
5. Bake for approximately 25–35 minutes. I like to leave a little crunch in the apple. Enjoy! ♥

Glazed Fruit Tart

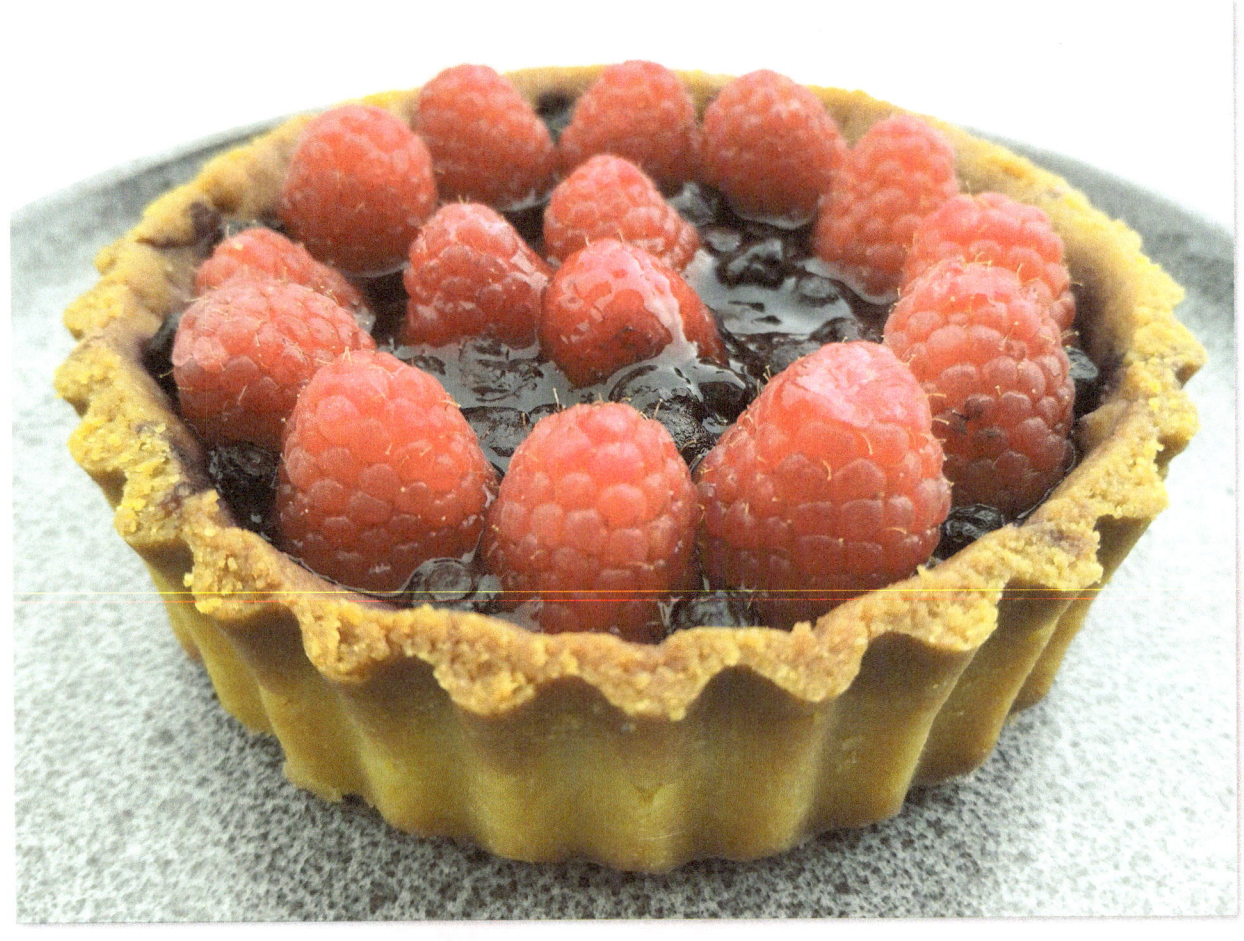

These little fruit custard tarts are incredibly cute and very tasty. I chose blueberries and raspberries, but you decide. I have based the macros on these two berries.

You don't have to add the jelly glaze. If you do and have any left over, just pour it into a pot for a little pudding later!

Equipment
- A bullet, hand blender, food processor or hand whisk
- Rolling pin
- 20 cm spring-based tin or 12-portion muffin tray (You can either make this as one big tart or 12 individual portions.)

Top Tips
- This is lovely served with double cream.
- This **cannot** be frozen.

Making Time
Approximately 25 minutes

Makes
12 portions

Per Portion
3.9g carbs / 5.2g protein / 187 calories / 16.4g fat

INGREDIENTS

The Base Recipe
- 1 batch custard tart (page 82) (**Please note that you will need to make up all of the pastry but only half of the custard filling, as this will be topped up with other ingredients.**)

The Rest of the Ingredients
- 1 packet sugar-free raspberry jelly
- 150ml boiling water
- 100ml cold water
- 100g raspberries
- 100g blueberries

METHOD

The Base Recipe
1. Make the custard tart (page 82)

Now the Final Parts of the Recipe
2. To make up the jelly, add the jelly crystals to the boiling water and stir until completely dissolved. Now stir in the cold water and pop in the fridge until the custard tart is cooked and completely cooled.
3. Layer the berries on top of the custard. Either you could pop them on in a stylish heap or go super pretty!
4. Pour the cold, starting-to-set jelly all over the berries and allow to set. This will take about an hour or so in the fridge, (don't feel that you have to use all of the jelly). Enjoy! ♥

Manchester Tart

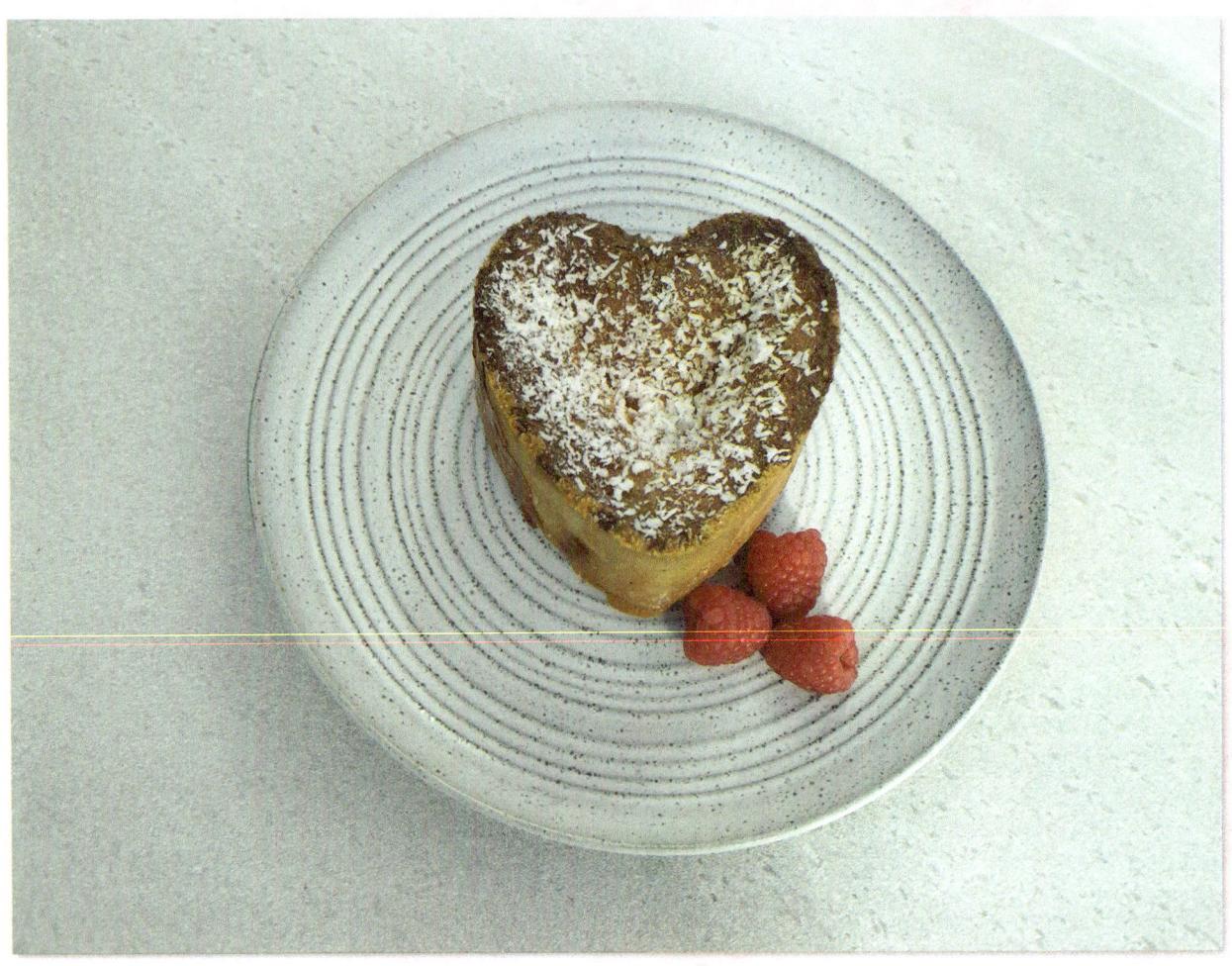

I was asked to come up with a low-carb version of this classic 1980s school-dinner pudding. This actually came first, then the custard tart base followed. It's a delightful pudding and well worth the effort.

Equipment
- Small non-stick saucepan
- Nutribullet, hand blender or food processor
- Rolling pin
- 8-inch spring-based tin or 12-portion muffin tray (You can either make this as one big tart or 12 individual portions.)

Top Tips
- This can be frozen.

Making Time
Approximately 45 minutes

Makes
12 portions

Per Portion
4 g carbs / 6.1 g protein / 234 calories / 21.2 g fat

INGREDIENTS

The Base Recipe
- 1 batch custard tart (page 82)

The Rest of the Ingredients
Jam
- 100g raspberries
- 5g Truvia sweetener (You might need extra sweetener for this if you don't like your fruit with a bit of tartness. I actually prefer it tart!)

Extras
- 30g desiccated coconut (15g for the jam layer and 15g for the final topping)

METHOD

The Base Recipe
1. Make the custard tart (page 82) and complete just the pastry part first and then pop back here for the jam making.

The Jam
2. Pop the berries, sweetener and a tiny dash of water into a small non-stick pan. Cook over a medium heat for 10–15 minutes, or until the berries have turned into a lovely silky jam and the juices have thickened, stirring occasionally.
3. Once the base is cooked, mix the jam and mash any large berries or whiz up in the food processor, then pour this on top of the base.
4. Sprinkle roughly **half** of the desiccated coconut over the jam.

The Custard Filling
5. Now pop back to the custard tart base (page 82) for the custard filling, but before you cook it, sprinkle the top with the remainder of the desiccated coconut. Enjoy! ♥

Wraps and Sauces

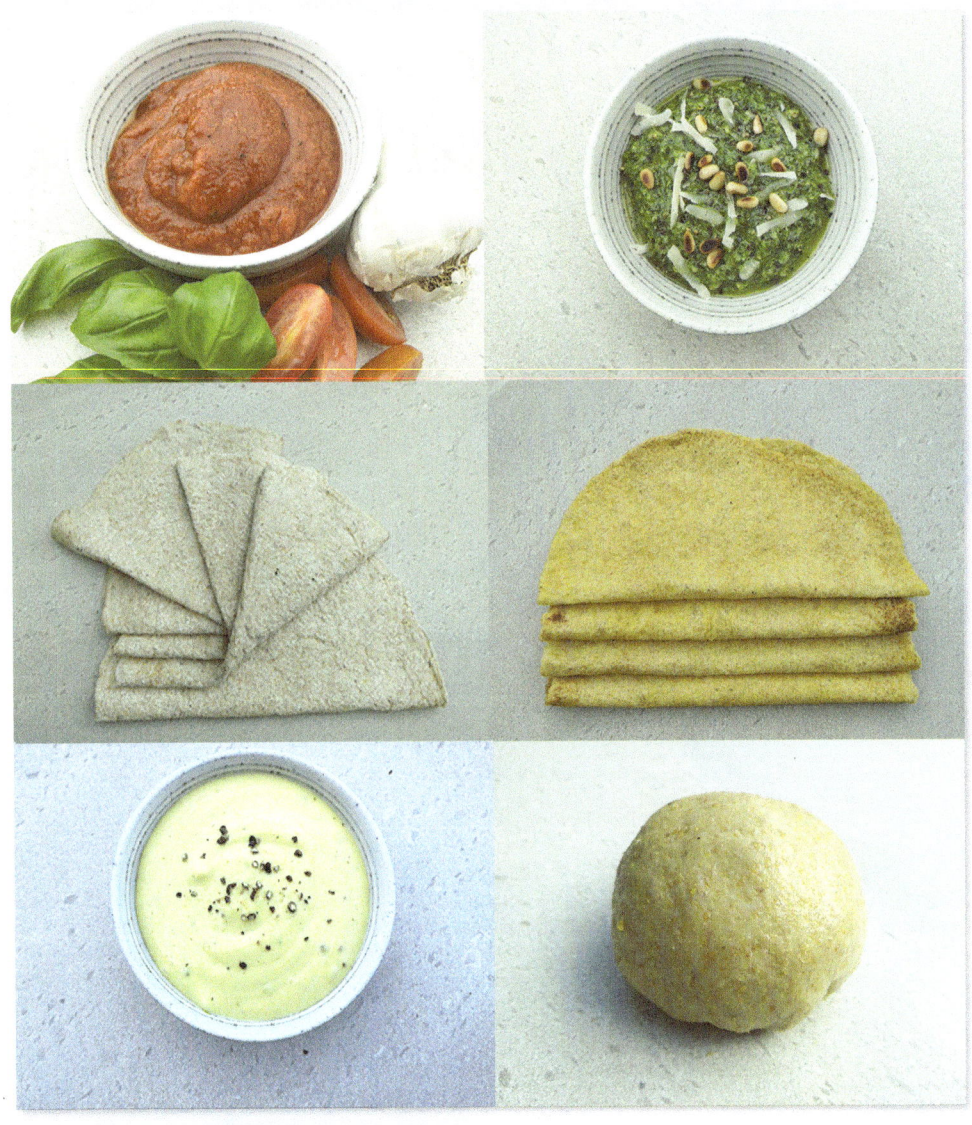

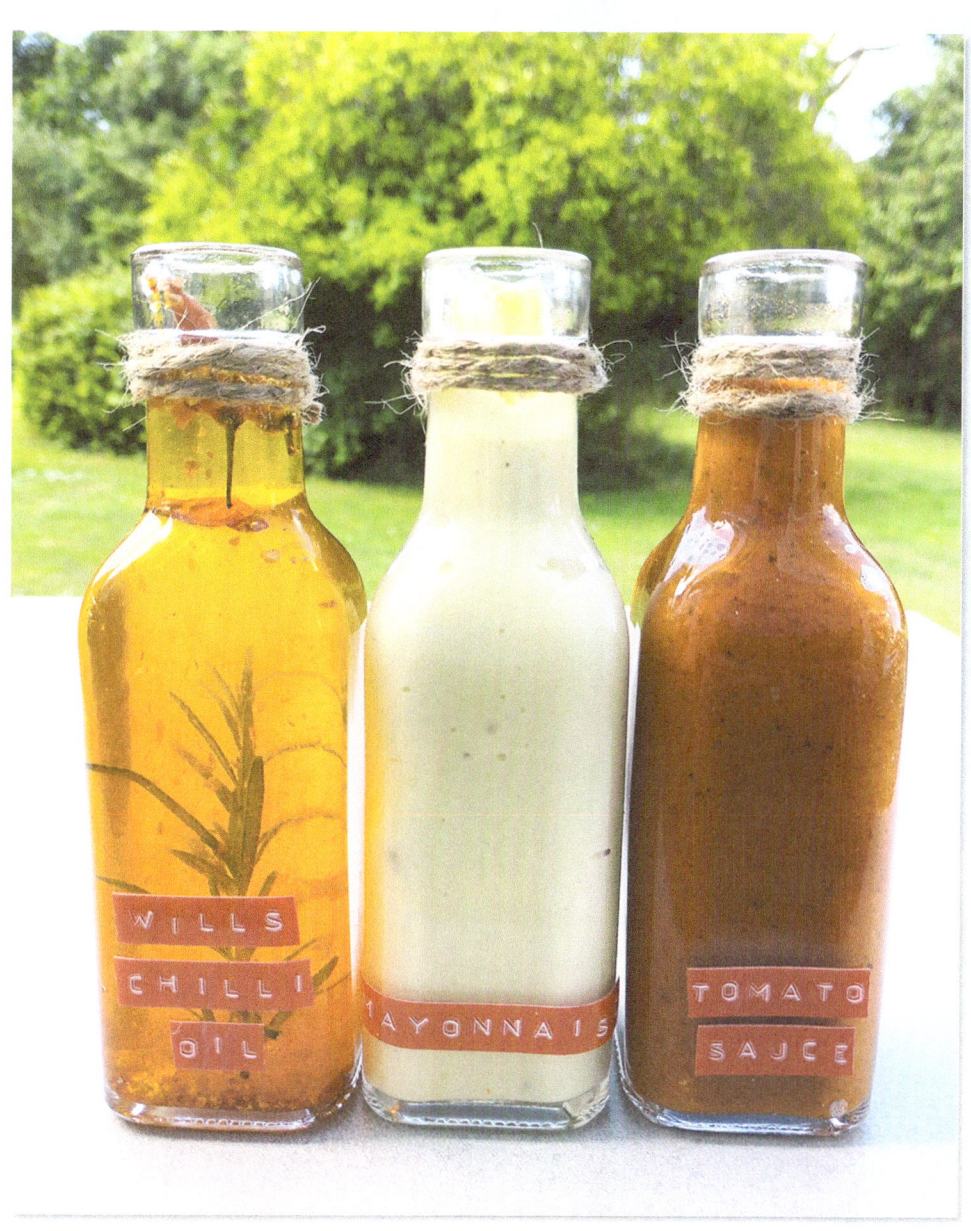

Bamboo Wraps

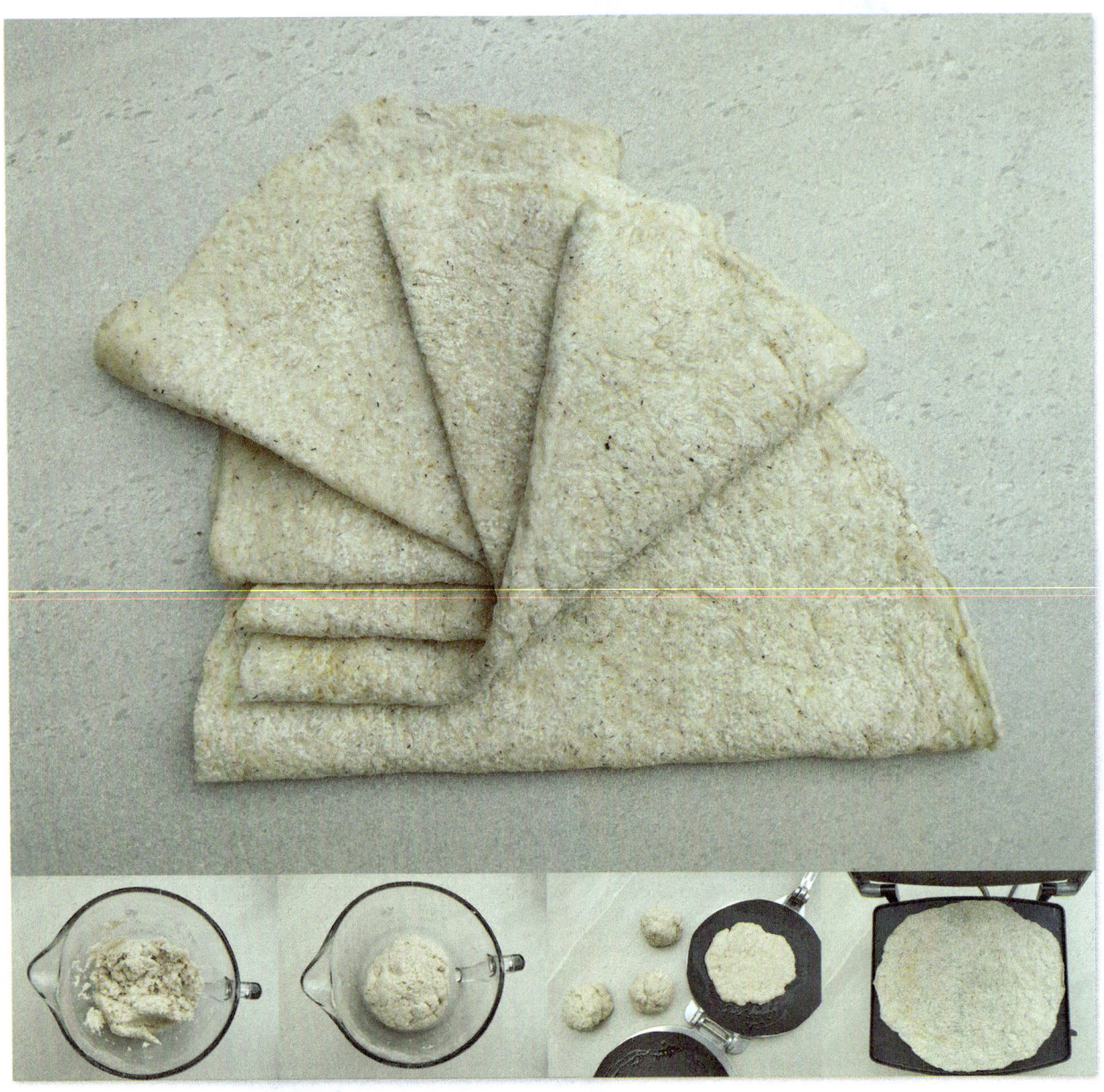

I do hope you like this recipe. This is Peter's favourite. It's super easy to make, especially if you have the two gadgets which are listed on the next page. If not, you can still do it old school and use a rolling pin and a frying pan.

Wraps and Sauces

Equipment

- Panini press and tortilla press (details about these on (page xv)
  If you don't have the above gadgets, you'll need:
- Rolling pin
- Silicone paper (page xvi)
- Good-quality, large non-stick frying pan

Top Tips

- Wet hands when handling this dough.
- This **can** be frozen.

Prep Time

Approximately 7 minutes with gadgets
Approximately 15 minutes without gadgets

Cook Time

Approximately 1½ minutes per wrap with gadgets
Approximately 3–4 minutes per wrap without gadgets

Makes

4 portions

Per Portion

0.3g carbs / 0.2g protein / 55 calories / 2.3g fat

INGREDIENTS

- 50g bamboo flour
- 8 level teaspoons (20 g) psyllium husk
- ½ teaspoon salt
- 280ml warm water
- 2 teaspoons (10 g) olive oil

NOTE TO CHEF When you've cooked your wraps, if they are a little stiff or crispy, after 5 minutes or so they will relax and soften, ready to roll or fold. Also, all flour qualities are different, so if you find that your dough, when cooked, goes a little like a paper doily, next time reduce the water by 10ml and try again.

METHOD

1. Add all the dry ingredients to a large bowl and mix.
2. Now add the warm water and olive oil.
3. Mix well with a spoon or spatula for about 20 seconds or until well mixed.
4. Scrape the dough into a nice tidy ball.
5. Leave to rest for 5 minutes. **This is so the psyllium husk can soak up the water. Trust the process!**

If you are using the two gadgets

1. Switch on your panini press, then line and grease your tortilla press so the dough slides as you press it (I use olive oil).
2. Wet your hands.
3. Divide your dough into four equal balls.
4. Pop one ball in the centre of the tortilla press, and press.
5. Now oil your panini press.
6. Pop your circular dough in the centre of the hot panini press. Close the lid and cook for 90 seconds. If you'd like a larger wrap, then after 20 seconds of cooking, hold the lid down a little firmly for 10 seconds (I pop a tea towel on top to stop myself getting burnt), then release the pressure and carry on cooking for a further minute, but still with the lid closed.
7. Pop onto a plate while you move on to the next wrap. Enjoy! ♥

If you are making these by hand

1. Wet your hands.
2. Divide your dough into four equal balls.
3. Grease your rolling pin with olive oil.
4. Roll out onto a silicone rolling mat (page xvi) or greaseproof paper. Grease everything. You may find it easier between two sheets of greaseproof or silicone paper. Go as large and as thin as you possibly dare, as it may shrink a little in the cooking process.
5. Heat up your pan with a little olive oil.
6. Transfer to the hot pan. Do this ever so carefully, as it's delicate at this stage, and if the wrap folds as you pop it in the pan, you can't fix it—although you can quickly pull it out and re-roll if you're super quick!
7. Now the next bit will depend on your pan and hob. I cooked for 90–120 seconds on the first side and then less than 60 seconds on the reverse side.
8. And that's it! Enjoy! ♥

Lupin Wraps

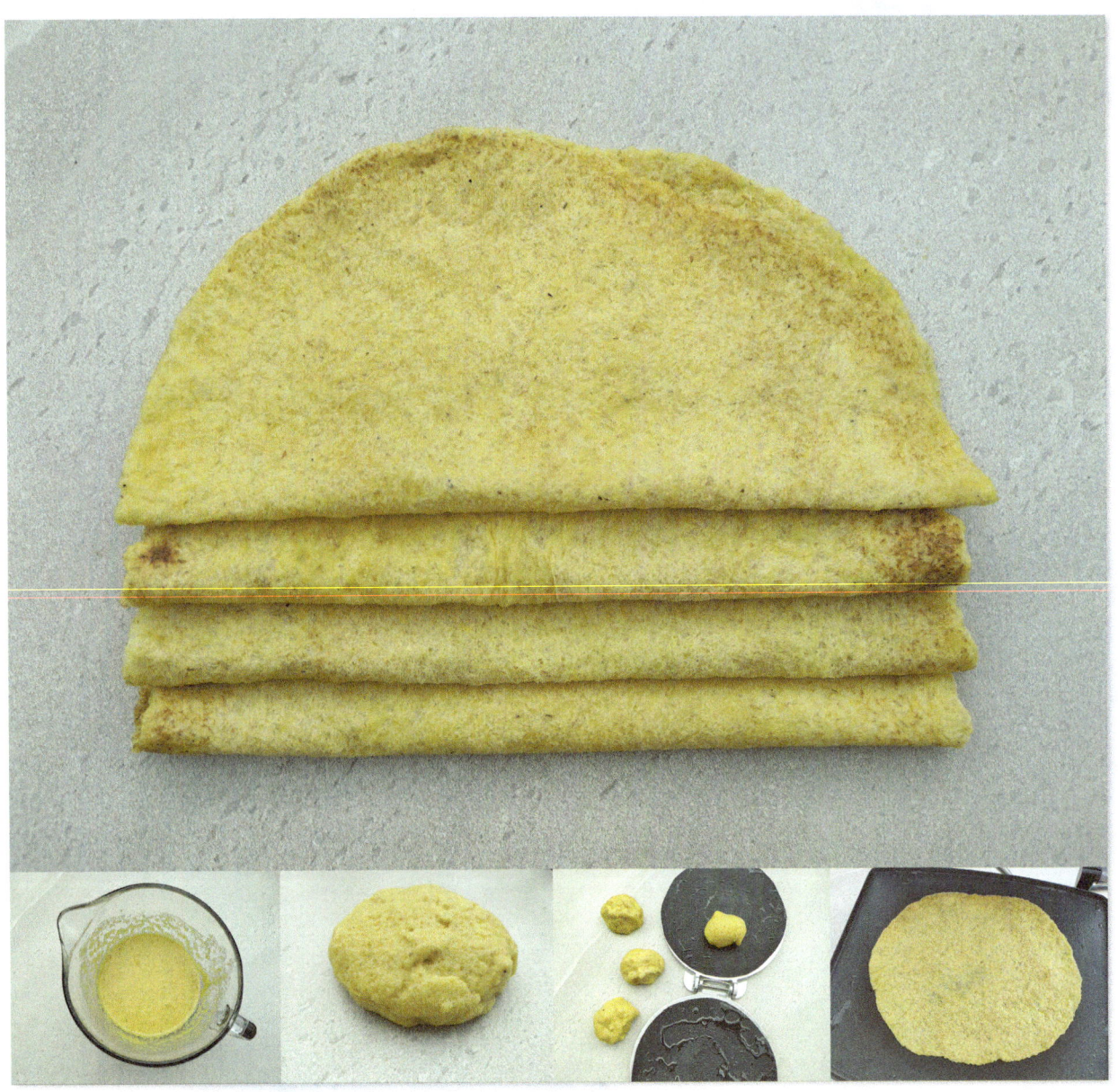

I do hope you like this recipe. This is my favourite. It's super easy to make, especially if you have the two gadgets which are listed on the next page. If not, you can still do it old school and use a rolling pin and a frying pan.

Equipment
- Panini press and tortilla press (details about these on (page xv)
  If you don't have the above gadgets, you'll need:
- Rolling pin
- Silicone paper (page xvi)
- Good-quality, large non-stick frying pan

Top Tips
- Wet hands when handling this dough.
- This **can** be frozen.

Prep Time
Approximately 7 minutes with gadgets
Approximately 15 minutes without gadgets

Cooking Time
Approximately 1½ minutes per wrap with gadgets
Approximately 3–4 minutes per wrap without gadgets

Makes 4 portions

Per Portion
2g carbs / 5.9g protein / 77 calories / 3.7g fat

INGREDIENTS
- 50g lupin flour
- 8 level teaspoons (20 g) psyllium husk
- ½ teaspoon salt
- 190g warm water
- 2 teaspoons (10 g) olive oil

NOTE TO CHEF When you've cooked your wraps, if they are a little stiff or crispy, after 5 minutes or so they will relax and soften, ready to roll or fold. Also, all flour qualities are different, so if you find that your dough, when cooked, goes a little like a paper doily, next time reduce the water by 10ml and try again.

METHOD
1. Add all the dry ingredients to a large bowl and mix.
2. Now add the warm water and olive oil.
3. Mix well with a spoon or spatula for about 20 seconds or until well mixed.
4. Scrape the dough into a nice tidy ball.
5. Leave to rest for 5 minutes. **This is so the psyllium husk can soak up the water. Trust the process!**

If you are using the two gadgets
1. Switch on your panini press. Line and grease your tortilla press so the dough slides as you press it (I use olive oil).
2. Wet your hands
3. Divide your dough into four equal balls.
4. Pop one ball in the centre of the tortilla press, and press.
5. Now oil your panini press.
6. Pop your circular dough in the centre of the hot panini press. Close the lid and cook for 90 seconds. If you'd like a larger wrap, then after 20 seconds of cooking, hold the lid down a little firmly for 10 seconds (I pop a tea towel on top to stop myself getting burnt), then release the pressure and carry on cooking for a further minute, but still with the lid closed.
7. Pop onto a plate while you move on to the next wrap. Enjoy! ♥

If you are making these by hand
1. Wet your hands.
2. Divide your dough into four equal balls.
3. Grease your rolling pin with olive oil.
4. Roll out onto a silicone rolling mat (page xvi) or greaseproof paper. Grease everything. You may find it easier between two sheets of greaseproof or silicone paper. Go as large and as thin as you possibly dare, as it may shrink a little in the cooking process.
5. Heat up your pan with a little olive oil.
6. Transfer to the hot pan. Do this ever so carefully, as it's delicate at this stage, and if the wrap folds as you pop it in the pan, you can't fix it—although you can quickly pull it out and re-roll it if you're super quick!
7. Now, the next bit will depend on your pan and hob. I cooked for 90–120 seconds on the first side and then less than 60 seconds on the reverse side.
8. And that's it! Enjoy! ♥

MKD (Michele's Keto Dough)

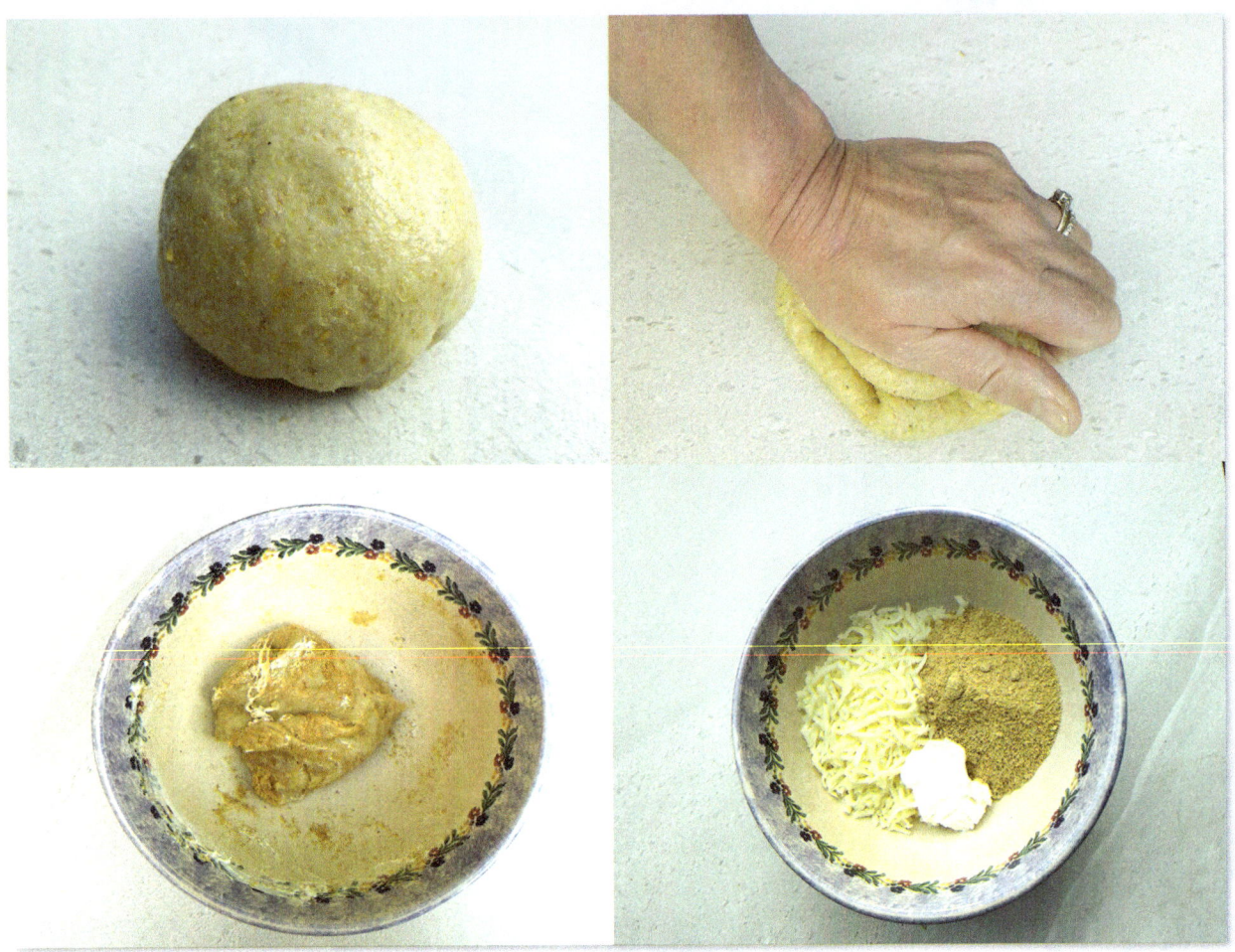

This is a very versatile dough and makes a wonderful pizza base. Equally, a very filling alternative lasagne sheet (page 10). It's very quick to make, about 90 seconds in the microwave and then just roll and bake.

Equipment
- Large microwave bowl
- Greaseproof paper
- Rolling pin

Top Tip
- This **can** be frozen.

Making Time
1–2 minutes in the microwave then approximately 10–15 minutes in the oven

Whole Recipe
10.4g carbs / 57.2g protein / 1010 calories / 81.1g fat (*if using ground almonds*)

9.8g carbs / 58.6g protein / 909 calories / 66.5g fat (*if using milled linseed*)

INGREDIENTS
- 170g ready-grated mozzarella (the mozzarella balls **can't** be used for this recipe)
- 70g milled linseed, but you can also use ground almonds or other mixed seeds
- 30g cream cheese
- ½ teaspoon salt

METHOD
1. Heat the oven to 180°C or the Ninja to 170°C.
2. Add all the ingredients to a large microwave bowl.
3. Microwave on full power for about 90 seconds. When the mozzarella has melted, it's ready to stir.
4. If it's not quite ready, return to the microwave and heat through for a further 20 seconds.
5. Give it a stir until it becomes a lovely smooth dough.
6. Work this dough while it's still hot.
7. Roll out the dough to the size of your lasagne dish and bake for approximately for 15 minutes or until light brown and crispy.
8. Now back to the lasagne on page 10.

NOTE TO CHEF If for any reason you can't roll out immediately, when you are ready, pop it back in the microwave for about 10 seconds and roll out immediately. This dough is very forgiving. Also, this doesn't need to fit perfectly. Once cooked, just break it up to fit your dish, just like lasagne.

You Can Also Use This to Make Pizza Bases
1. Once rolled out, I like to cook for 5 minutes on the one side, without any toppings first.
2. Then I flip it over and pop the toppings on.
3. Bake for a further 10 minutes or so. Enjoy! ♥

Pesto

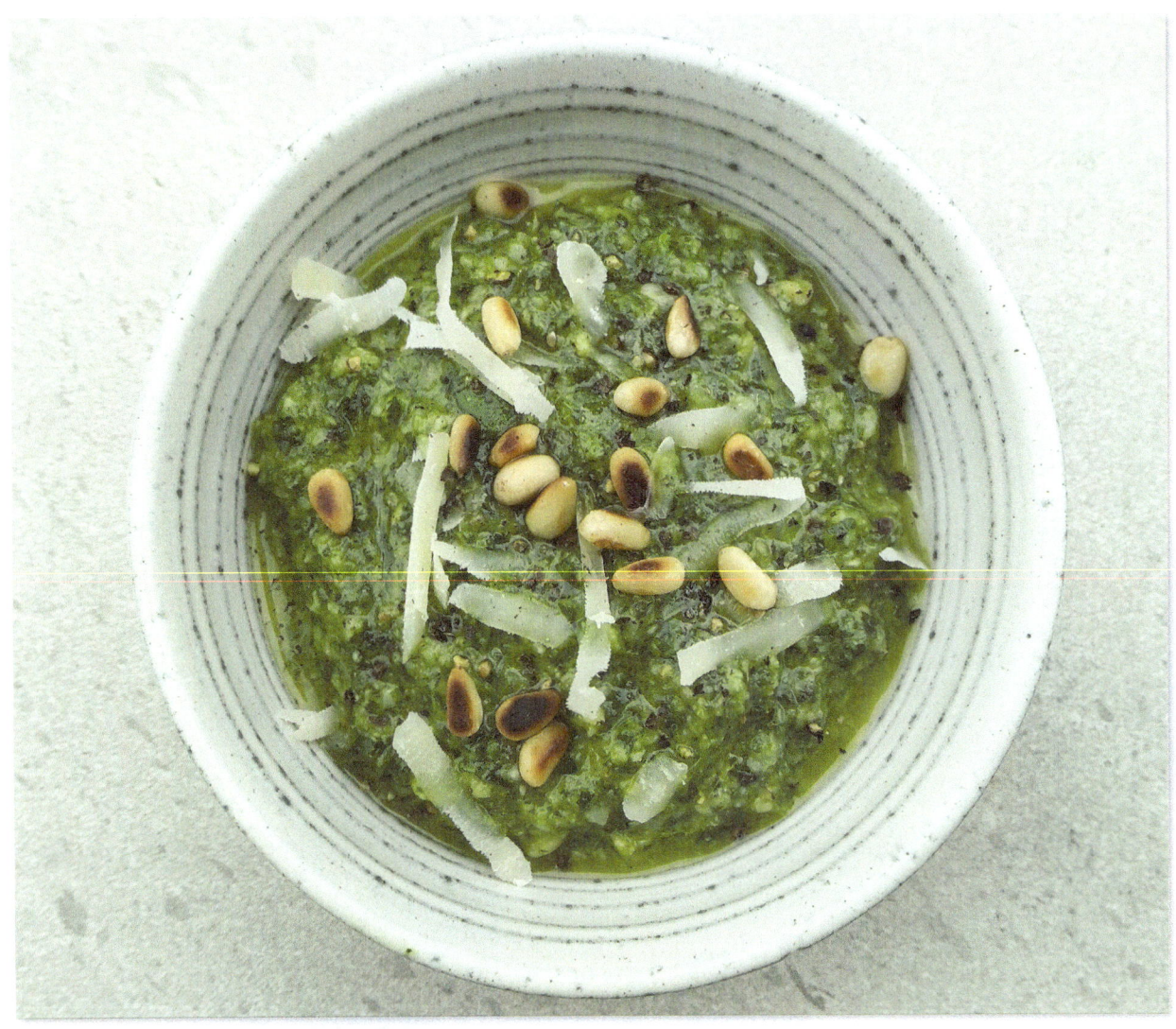

This pesto is used in the yorkshire pudding section, (page 78). But what else could you use it for? Pesto topped chicken, Cream cheese and pesto Salmon, Creme Fraiche and pesto dip or stirred through some roasted vegetables. Or just keep it in a jar in the fridge and spread it on some low carb toast.

Equipment
- A small non-stick saucepan or frying pan
- Hand blender or small food processor (page xvi)
- Storage jar (page xv)

Top Tips
- This will keep in the fridge for at least a week or so.
- You can also use walnuts.
- This **can** be frozen.

Making Time
Approximately 10 minutes

Whole Recipe
4.3g carbs / 14.4g protein / 915 calories / 93.8g fat

INGREDIENTS
- 25g pine nuts
- 50g fresh basil (You can swap for another fresh herb of choice — coriander is lovely too, parsley, or spinach.)
- 25g grated parmesan
- 75ml olive oil
- ¾ teaspoon garlic puree or 1 garlic clove
- Salt and pepper, season to taste

METHOD
1. Heat a small pan and add the pine nuts to toast them until golden. This will take about 2 minutes.
2. Next add the browned pine nuts and all the remaining ingredients to a small food processor (page xvi) and blitz until smooth.
3. Season to taste.
4. Transfer to a small airtight container (page xv). Enjoy! ♥

Mayonnaise

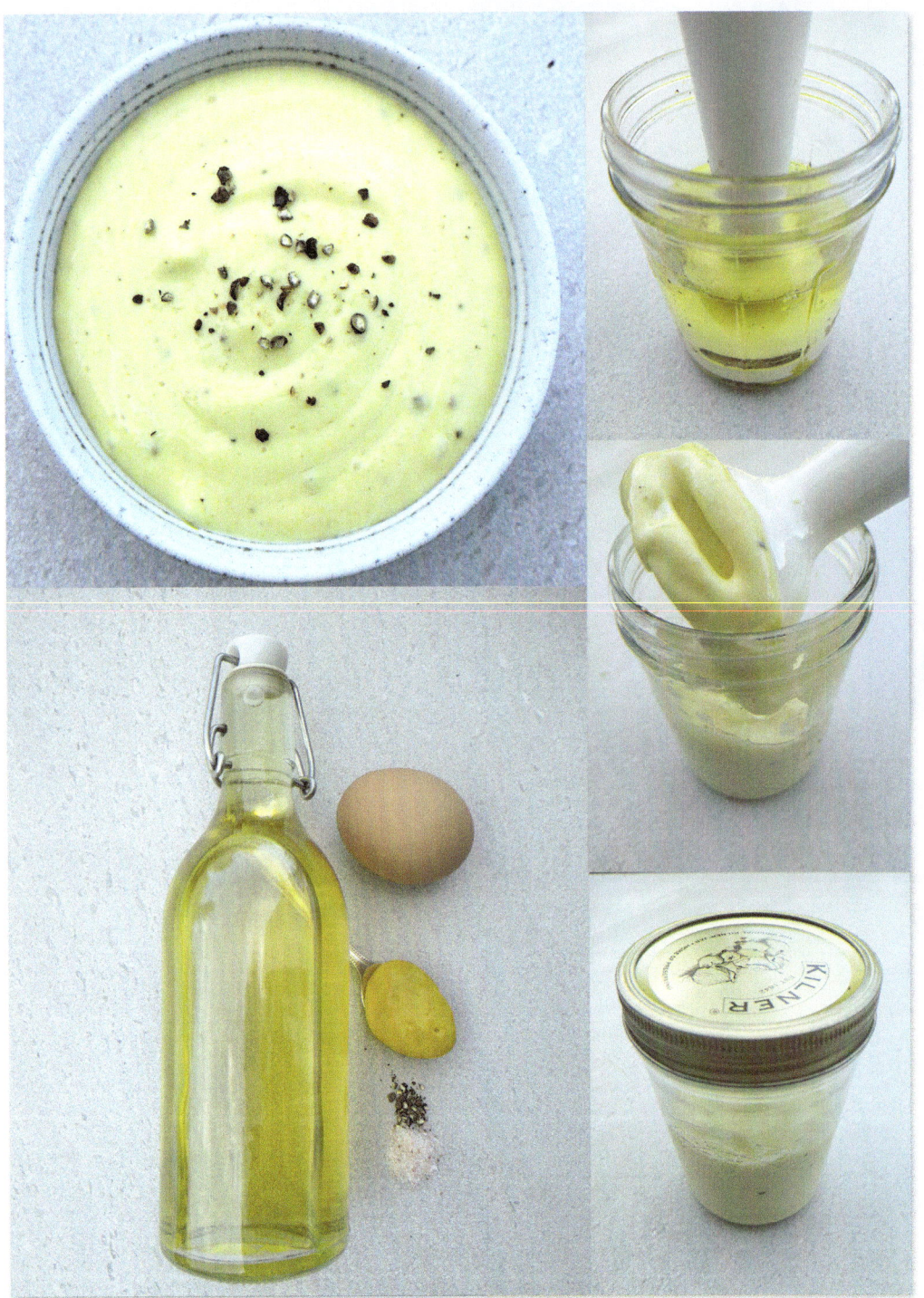

This is a great little recipe that is so unbelievably easy to make. You can change the flavour by swapping the mustard for horse raddish or fresh lemon juice.

Equipment
- Hand blender (page xvi)
- Tall, flat-bottomed, narrow jug, or you can mix it straight into a storage jar (page xv). (This saves on washing up; just make sure that the head of the blender fits right to the bottom of the jar.)

Top Tips
- This can be stored in the fridge for about a week, as long as the eggs are fresh.
- This recipe works every time for me, as long as I use a hand blender. It can be hit or miss if I use a food processor.
- This **cannot** be frozen.

Making Time
Approximately 3 minutes

Whole Recipe
0.1g carbs / 6.5g protein / 1099 calories / 119.1g fat

15g or 1 level tablespoon
0.0g carbs / 0.5g protein / 92 calories / 9.9g fat

INGREDIENTS
- 125g light or mild olive oil (using the light leaves a less bitter taste, but it's personal preference)
- 1 medium egg
- 1 heaped teaspoon Dijon mustard (I actually prefer 2 teaspoons wholegrain mustard)
- ¼ teaspoon salt
- ⅛ teaspoon freshly ground black pepper

METHOD
1. In a tall jug or size-appropriate storage jar, add the oil and then all the other ingredients.
2. Put the stick blender right to the base of the jug and blend.
3. As it thickens, gently move the blender up to the top of the oil so all the ingredients are blended.
4. All of this takes no more than 10 seconds.
5. Done. Enjoy! ♥

Tomato Sauce

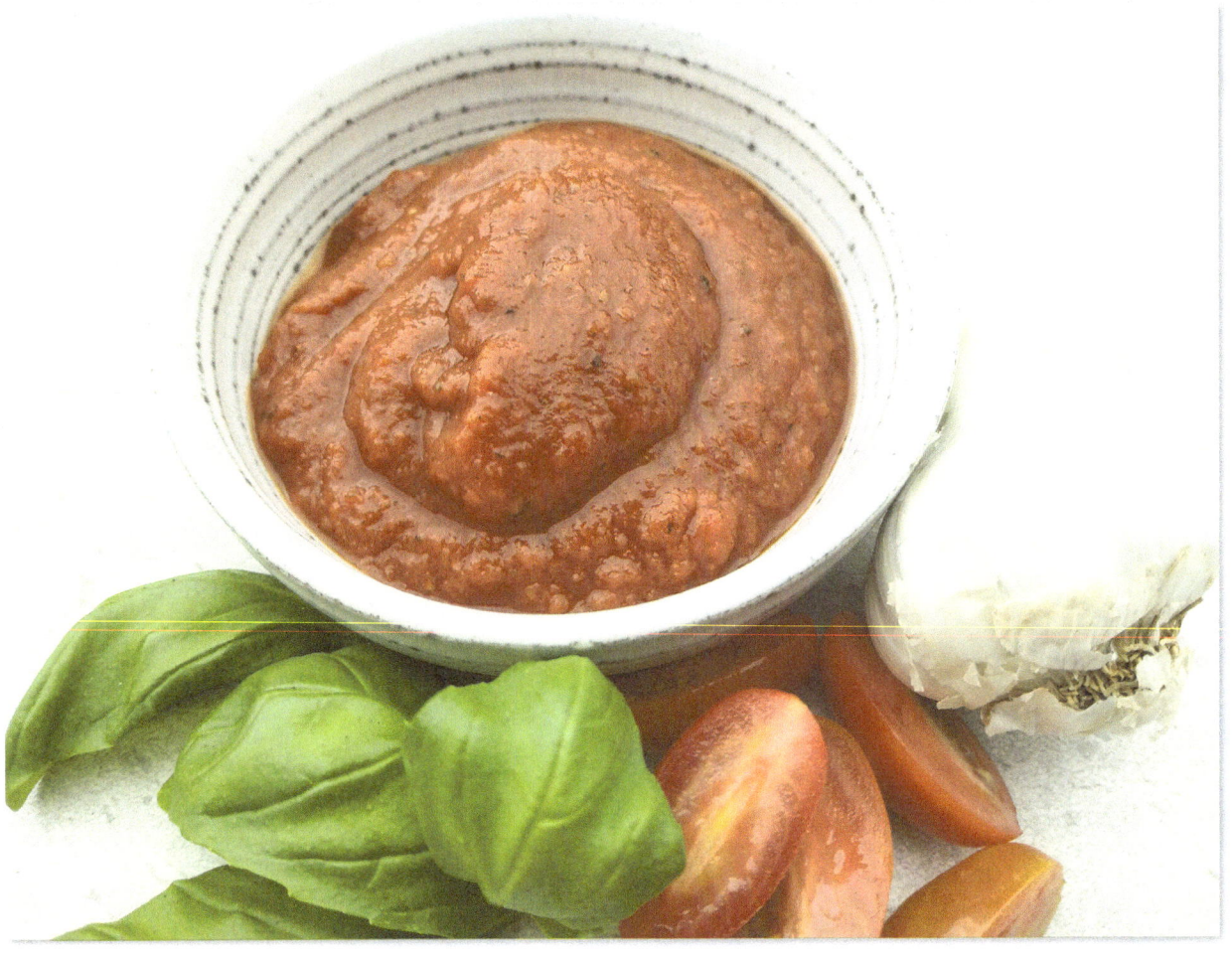

This is a really useful sauce to have in the fridge, whether it's a ketchup or a pizza sauce. It should keep for at least a couple of weeks in a sealed container (page xv).

Equipment
- Hand blender (page xvi) or a bullet
- Small non-stick saucepan

Top Tips
- This **can** be stored in the fridge for at least a week or more in a sealed container (page xv).
- This **can** be frozen.

Making Time
Approximately 15 minutes

Whole Recipe
27g carbs / 8.7g protein / 315 calories / 19.7g fat

15g or 1 level tablespoon
0.8g carbs / 0.2g protein / 9 calories / 0.6g fat

INGREDIENTS
- 400g tinned tomatoes
- 60g tomato puree
- 40g shallots or 50g red onions, roughly chopped
- 20g olive oil
- 1½ teaspoons paprika
- 1 teaspoon dried oregano or a handful of fresh basil
- 1 teaspoon Truvia sweetener
- ¾ teaspoon garlic puree or 1 garlic clove
- ¾ teaspoon salt
- ¼ teaspoon freshly ground black pepper

METHOD
1. Put all your sauce ingredients into a Bullet, or use a hand blender, and blitz until smooth.
2. Transfer to a small saucepan.
3. Heat up until bubbling and simmer for about 10 minutes to reduce the sauce.
4. Add extra seasoning or sweetener to taste.
5. This can be stored in the fridge for at least a week, or more in a sealed container (page xv). Enjoy! ♥

Will's Chilli Oil

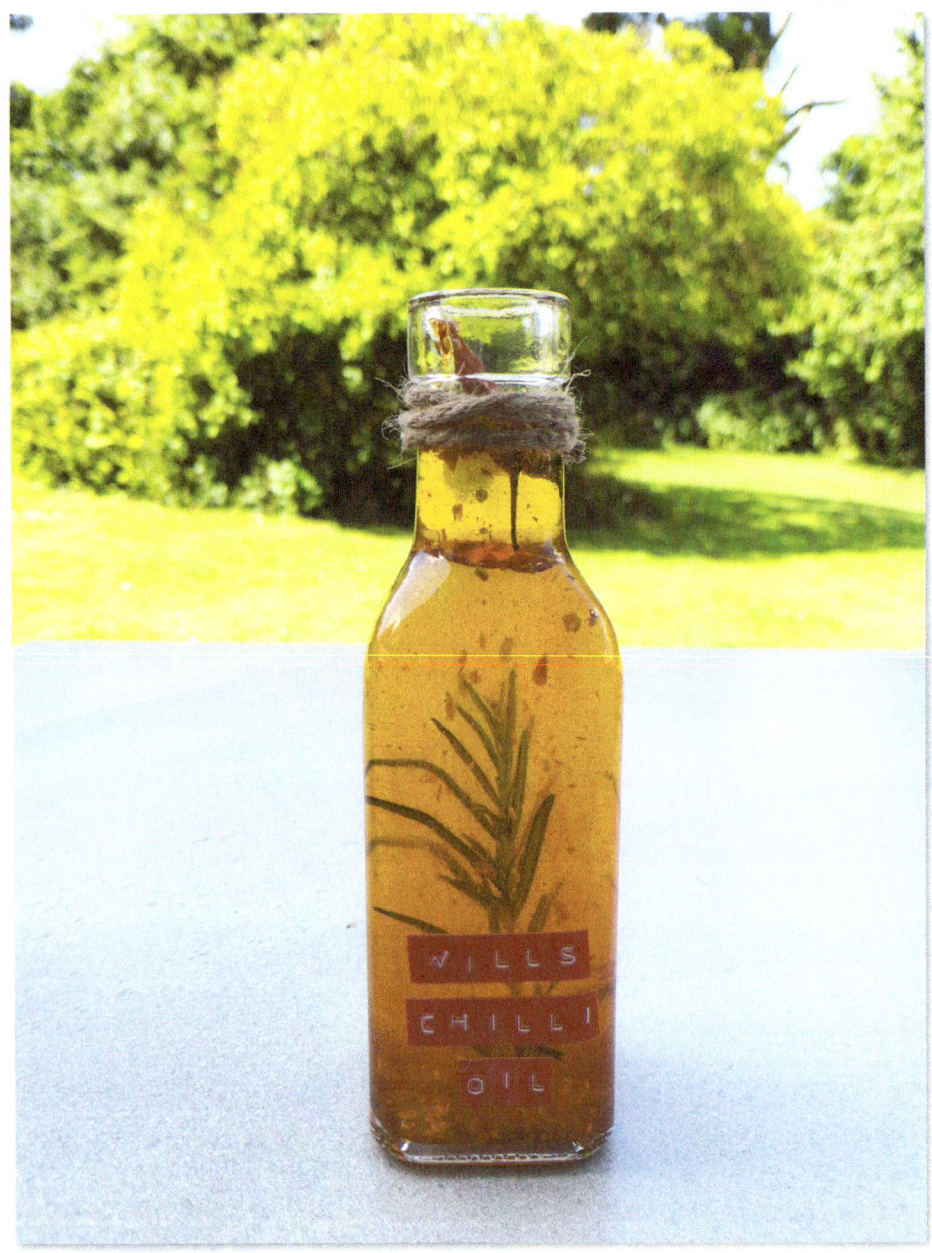

This is a particular oil that I use lots in my day-to-day cooking. It's instantly full of flavour. My son made it for me with his home-grown chilli (thank you, Will ♥), but not everyone has access to this, so chilli flakes or powder are fine too. The strength of the oil depends on the strength of your chilli. The chilli this time was called Basket of Fire, so you can imagine, this time it blew my head off! So, you decide, and also the strength of the chilli flavour intensifies as it matures. If it is too strong, you have two choices to rectify it: use less in the cooking, or water it down with more olive oil. I often top the oil up when it's getting low.

Equipment
- Approximately 300ml – 350ml bottle with a lid. Kitner bottles always work well. You could also use the bottle that the oil came in.
- Funnel

Top Tips
- This makes fabulous gifts.
- This **cannot** be frozen.

Making Time
Approximately 2 minutes

Whole Recipe
0.5g carbs / 0.3g protein / 2477 calories / 274.6g fat

15g or 1 level tablespoon
0.0g carbs / 0.0g protein / 134 calories / 13.7g fat

INGREDIENTS
- 5–10g dried chillies (either your own grown and dried or bought chilli flakes)
- ½ teaspoon Kashmiri spice
- 1 sprig rosemary (optional)
- 250–300ml olive oil

METHOD
1. Sterilise the bottle or jar.
2. Add all the dry ingredients first, then top up with the olive oil.
3. Give it a shake, and that's it!
4. Always shake the bottle before you use it (**Note to self: always make sure the lid is on tight!**)
5. The taste will mature over time. Enjoy! ♥

Index

Baked Enchiladas, Bolognese 4
Baked Vegetables and Chorizo, Salsa 54
Bamboo Wraps 94
Basil, Sundried Tomatoes and Feta Coleslaw 14
Beef and Leek in Gravy Pie 34
Biryani, Curry 26

Cheddar and Peanuts, Coleslaw 15
Chicken and Chorizo, Rainbow Rice 44
Chicken and Egg Soup 64
Chicken and Parmesan, Salsa 56
Chicken and Roast Pepper Curry 28
Chicken and Vegetable in Gravy Pie 36
Chicken, Tomato and Roasted Vegetable Curry 30
Chilli Bake, Bolognese 6
Chowder Soup 66
Cottage Pie, Bolognese 8
Creamy Chicken and Ham Pie 38
Curried Eggs, Coleslaw 16

Far Breton, Custard Tart 84
Festive Apple Crunch, Custard Tart 86
Fish Paella, Rainbow Rice 46

Glazed Fruit Tart, Custard Tart 88

Ham and Spring Onion, Quiche 20

Kedgeree, Rainbow Rice 48

Lamb and Leek, Yorkshire Pudding 74
Lasagne, Bolognese 10
Lupin Wraps 96

Manchester Tart, Custard Tart 90
Mayonnaise 102
Meatballs in a Tomato Sauce, Yorkshire Pudding 76
Minestrone Soup 68

MKD (Michele's Keto Dough) 98
My Kitchen Gadgets xv

Nutty Vegetarian, Rainbow Rice 50

One Bolognese Four Ways 2
One Coleslaw Four Ways 12
One Crustless Quiche Four Ways 18
One Curry Four Ways 24
One Custard Tart Four Ways 82
One Pie Crust Four Ways 32
One Rainbow Rice Four Ways 42
One Salsa Four Ways 52
One Soup Four Ways 62
One Yorkshire Pudding Four Ways 72

Pesto 100
Pesto and Goats Cheese, Yorkshire Pudding 78

Raspberry Popover, Yorkshire Pudding 80
Roasted Vegetable and Butter Bean Curry 29

Salmon and Green Vegetable Parcel, Salsa 58
Salmon, Broccoli and Dill, Quiche 21
Spinach and Feta Pie 40
Stilton and Mushroom, Quiche 22
Stilton and Walnut, and Optional Apple, Coleslaw 17
Substitutions xiii
Sun Dried Tomatoes, Feta and Spinach, Quiche 23

Tomato Sauce 104
Tortilla Chips and 3 Mexican Dips, Salsa 60

Vegetable Smooth and Creamy Soup 70

Will's Chilli Oil 106
Wraps and Sauces 92

Printed and bound by CPI Group (UK) Ltd, Croydon, CR0 4YY
15/03/2025
01833653-0003